KILLING
SEASON

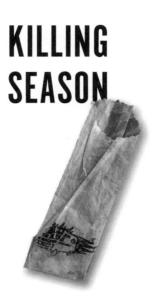

KILLING SEASON

A PARAMEDIC'S DISPATCHES

FROM THE FRONT LINES

OF THE

OPIOID EPIDEMIC

Peter Canning

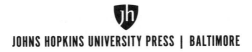

JOHNS HOPKINS UNIVERSITY PRESS | BALTIMORE

© 2021 Peter Canning
All rights reserved. Published 2021
Printed in the United States of America on acid-free paper
9 8 7 6 5 4 3 2 1

Johns Hopkins University Press
2715 North Charles Street
Baltimore, Maryland 21218-4363
www.press.jhu.edu

Library of Congress Cataloging-in-Publication Data

Names: Canning, Peter, 1958– author.
Title: Killing season : a paramedic's dispatches from the front lines
    of the opioid epidemic / Peter Canning.
Description: Baltimore : Johns Hopkins University Press, [2021] |
    Includes bibliographical references and index.
Identifiers: LCCN 2020013521 | ISBN 9781421439853 (hardcover) |
    ISBN 9781421439860 (ebook)
Subjects: LCSH: Canning, Peter, 1958– | Opioid abuse—Connecticut—Hartford. |
    Drug addicts—Medical care—Connecticut—Hartford. | Emergency medical
    services—Connecticut—Hartford.
Classification: LCC RC568.O45 C35 2021 | DDC 362.29/3097463—dc23
LC record available at https://lccn.loc.gov/2020013521

A catalog record for this book is available from the British Library.

Special discounts are available for bulk purchases of this book. For more information,
please contact Special Sales at specialsales@press.jhu.edu.

Johns Hopkins University Press uses environmentally friendly book materials,
including recycled text paper that is composed of at least 30 percent post-consumer
waste, whenever possible.

To my wife, Chevaughn, and our three children,
Ashley, Lauren, and Zoey, who bring me joy, pride, and
laughter, and who always welcome me home

How we respond to this crisis is a moral test for America. Are we a nation willing to take on an epidemic that is causing great human suffering and economic loss? Are we able to live up to that most fundamental obligation we have as human beings: to care for one another?

UNITED STATES SURGEON GENERAL VIVEK H. MURTHY,
2016 REPORT FACING ADDICTION IN AMERICA

Addiction is defined as a chronic, relapsing disorder characterized by compulsive drug seeking and use despite adverse consequences. It is considered a brain disorder, because it involves functional changes to brain circuits involved in reward, stress, and self-control, and those changes may last a long time after a person has stopped taking drugs.

NATIONAL INSTITUTE ON DRUG ABUSE

I'll die young, but it is like kissing God.

LENNY BRUCE ON SHOOTING HEROIN

CONTENTS

KILLING
SEASON

Introduction

My name is Peter Canning. I am a full-time paramedic in Hartford, Connecticut, an area hard hit by the opioid epidemic and, in particular, by the synthetic opioid fentanyl, which in the summer of 2017 was in 90 percent of the city's heroin supply. When I started as a paramedic on the streets of Hartford twenty-five years ago, I believed that drug users were victims only of their own character flaws. While I took care of them, I did not care for them. They were a scourge on the health care system and the community. They were junkies and deadbeats. They lacked personal responsibility, and their behavior was criminal. That's what I believed. Keep using drugs, I'd tell them, and you will end up dead or in jail, which many of them did.

Today, my views on drug users are different. As the overdoses escalated, I began asking my patients how they got started on their perilous journeys. While no two tales were the same, they shared unremitting similarities. Their entries into addiction—whether through legal drugs prescribed by their doctor following injury or illness, spare pills offered by a friend to help with nagging pain, or through experimentation, innocent or otherwise—spun them into tortuous futures they could not have foreseen and from which, for many, there was no escape. Over and over I heard "I used to be a normal person once." Their stories changed my view and moved me to educate myself about the science of addiction and, armed with that understanding, to fight against the stigmatization of users.

I know now that addiction is a chronic brain disease whose victims deserve our empathy, support, and kindness. I know that stigma—viewing and treating drug users as reprobates—does almost as much damage as the drugs do themselves to patients' ability to recover and heal. I know users are not riffraff, deadbeats, or scumbags; they are our brothers, sisters, parents, dear friends, neighbors, and members of our communities who got caught up in a storm not of their own making that continues to claim millions of victims nationwide and in other countries around the world. People addicted to opioids are victims of a disease in the same way that those who suffer from heart, lung, or other debilitating maladies and disabilities are victims of their disease. Worse yet, they are victims of an epidemic largely fueled by the ignorance of our medical establishment and by the greed of the pharmaceutical industry, which at times has done wonders for human health but, in this case, has betrayed its promise for the sake of obscene profits.

Today, rather than scorning or simply ignoring people's drug use, I embrace harm reduction, a strategy I had never heard of until just a few years ago when I listened to a remarkable man named Mark Jenkins speak at a conference. Harm reduction, as Mark told us that day, accepts that people are going to use drugs and works to minimize the negative consequences of their drug use. It recognizes that many people use drugs because drugs work for them, sparing them the horrible sickness of withdrawal and blunting the pain, both physical and mental, that the years and events in their lives have brought them. Mark emphasized that we have to help the living because dead people don't make good decisions. Harm reduction helps people stay alive until they are in a place where they are open to change and able to receive help.

Now, deputized into the harm reduction movement, I "meet people where they are," and I look at those who use illegal drugs without judgment. Instead of telling my patients who use to just say no, I offer them avenues to recovery. If they are not ready for treatment, I tell them how to use drugs safely. Don't use alone, I say. Do a tester shot if you've bought from a new dealer or have a new batch. Don't mix opioids with benzodiazepines, or benzos. Always have naloxone available. Call 911 if someone overdoses. I tell them where they can get clean needles and how to treat their skin to avoid abscesses. I warn them about dangerous heroin batches for sale on the street. I have, when posted in my ambulance in certain neighborhoods, even had people use within my sight, knowing that they were safe when I watched over them. Like Mark, I believe we can't just stand by and let people die.

Ever since I started as a paramedic in 1995, I have kept journals about the job and the patients I have encountered, often writing in the ambulance front seat in between 911 dispatches, always trying to make sense of what I am feeling and experiencing. I wrote this book so that others can hear the voices of my patients, see what I have seen at overdose scenes and their critical aftermaths, and learn that drug users are as normal as you or me before they encounter, through whatever means, the opioids that spiral their life out of control. The stories and people in this book are real. Some names and details have been altered to protect confidentiality.

I am hopeful that people will join me in fighting stigma, embracing harm reduction, and focusing our country and communities on saving and restoring lives, and in helping the lost find their way home.

Before I became a paramedic, I worked as a policy aide and speechwriter for United States senator and later governor of

Connecticut Lowell Weicker. He used to say that the mark of this country's greatness is not how it treats its best citizens but how it treats the sickest and most vulnerable ones. After more than two decades of providing emergency medical care on city streets, I believe his words even more today than I did then, when I worked in the halls of power. As a nation, each breathing day, we should renew and live by that American promise.

Prologue

A teenage girl waves frantically from the front steps for us to hurry. "My brother! My brother!" she cries. Carrying my paramedic house bag and heart monitor, I run across the manicured lawn, up three marbled steps, and in through the front door. She motions me up the stairs toward the second floor. Framed family photos—camping trips, the beach, sporting events—line the stairwell. At the end of the hall, a bedroom door is open. A woman in a yellow dress, her back to me, is on her knees doing CPR. I toss my bag on the New York Giants bedspread and set my cardiac monitor down by the young man's head. He is lifeless, his face white with a blue tinge. I apply the defibrillator pads to his hairless chest. On his shoulder is a surgical scar. A 1 cc syringe lies on the carpet next to his left arm.

"Stop CPR," I say.

The heart monitor shows only a flatline—no sign of a heartbeat.

A police officer, who has arrived just behind us, eases away the mother, her makeup ruined by tears, as my partner puts his hands on the young man's chest. Watching a parent do CPR on her child is heartbreaking, and unfortunately, with this opioid scourge upon us, it is no longer an uncommon occurrence.

"Continue CPR."

Opioids, whether prescription drugs such as OxyContin or the illicit drug heroin, bind to multiple receptors in the brain. In the brain's reward center, opioids attach to receptors and trigger a release of dopamine, the chemical that produces pleasure. But in the brain stem, opioids attach to receptors that control breathing. When the opioids get a firm enough hold on these receptors, the user's respirations will slow to a critical level and sometimes stop altogether. People die of heroin overdoses from a lack of oxygen to the brain. That is what's happening here. We hope we can pull him back from the edge before it's too late.

The mother stands with her hand over her mouth, trembling. And we do what we can for her child. I take out an Ambu bag, a plastic face mask attached to a squeezable bag. With my left hand, my fingers under his jaw, my thumb above his nose, I hold the mask tightly sealed against his face and tilt his head back. I squeeze the bag with my right hand and watch his chest rise as air enters his lungs. Naloxone, the overdose antidote, is of no use at this late point. We have to get his heart going. While an arriving firefighter takes over the bagging, I insert a 14-gauge IV catheter into the external jugular vein in the young man's neck, attach to it a saline lock (to keep the IV clear), and push a milligram of epinephrine into his vein. Epinephrine, a pure stimulant, is his best hope.

"He's been out of rehab for six weeks and has been clean," his mother tells the officer. "He was doing really well. He said goodnight when he came home last night. We thought about checking on him, but we wanted to show him we trusted him. He didn't come down for breakfast when I called."

I can't help but look around the neatly ordered room: the bookshelf with wrestling trophies, the bright aquarium with impassive angelfish, the clothes hung in the open closet, the computer with a screen saver of a smiling young man and pretty red-haired girlfriend in prom attire. I can smell the bacon from the kitchen.

We stop for the next rhythm check. He is still flatline, and we go right back to CPR. A second responding police officer goes through the trash can by the bed. "Got 'em," he says. He holds up three small glassine envelopes: Killing Season. The wax-paper heroin bags are printed with the brand name and a menacing skull. Each bag had contained 0.1 gram of powder before the young man dumped it into his spoon, or cooker. I used to find it hard to believe that such a tiny amount of powder could wreak so much tragedy. But scenes as this are no longer new to us.

I wonder if the young man bought from his usual dealer or maybe from someone new. Did he ask for this brand with the grim skull on the bag? Was this a bad batch with a hot spot of fentanyl, the deadly synthetic opioid fifty times stronger than heroin that dealers are lacing their heroin with for extra strength? Or maybe he hadn't used for a while, trying to stay clean. His tolerance down, maybe he did the same amount he used to before he stopped, and it was too much for him. I wonder if he felt a warm, thrilling rush of pleasure when he pushed down the plunger. Did he gently fade away, or did he suddenly seize with a violent jerk, unable to expand his lungs to breathe, panic filling his last moments?

We work him. I give another shot of epinephrine five minutes after the first. Vomit comes from his mouth now, a byproduct of the CPR. We tilt him to the side, to prevent him from drawing it into his lungs. When his throat is clear, I lay him back. I insert my laryngoscope blade into his mouth, its tiny light bulb illuminating my view. The blade doesn't cut; it pushes the tongue aside. I suction his airway until I can see his vocal cords. I slide a plastic endotracheal tube into his mouth, still keeping his tongue out of the way with the blade. I slide the tube through the cords and then, with a syringe, blow up the small-cuffed balloon that seals the tube against the walls of his trachea so that we can ventilate him better.

His mother stands by the closet door, watching us, helpless. "Come here," I say. "Come hold his hand." I make space for her to kneel by his side. "Talk to him."

When I was a newer medic, I liked to keep the family away, but after twenty-five years of this, I think it is better to have the family present during a resuscitation attempt. No one should be alone as he departs this world.

"Come on, my baby. Don't leave me." She cries and kisses his hand.

His sister kneels next to her mother, holding her, and shouting: "Come on, Johnny! Fight! Fight!"

I give a fourth epinephrine. Moments later his exhaled carbon dioxide reading on my monitor jumps from 24 to 61—a sign we may have restarted his heart. "Stop CPR!" I say. I feel his neck. His carotid artery throbs. "I've got a pulse. Let's get his blood pressure."

"Yes, baby!" his mother cries.

"We have his heart back," I caution, "but he's been down a long time."

My partner slips the blood pressure cuff around the young man's arm. I continue to squeeze the Ambu bag. No sign yet of spontaneous respiration. I check his pupils. They are still fixed and dilated. I fear the epinephrine has merely restarted his heart, and the damage to his brain from being without oxygen so long is likely permanent.

"Come on, baby," his mother says. "Open your eyes! Open your eyes for me! Let me see you again!"

We secure him to a board with straps around his calves and waist and crisscrossed around his chest, with a thick strap across his head. We tie his hands together with kling bandages to keep his limp arms from falling off the board when we carry him. I continue ventilating throughout. His heart rate has come down as the epinephrine is wearing off. His concentration of exhaled carbon dioxide is now holding in a normal range.

I detach the Ambu bag for the carry down. Because I am taller than my partner, I take the bottom end, while he holds the top. A firefighter has his hand on my back to keep me from falling as I step backward, leaning my shoulder against the wall for support. I accidently knock a photograph off the wall and hear it tumble down the stairs, the glass breaking. I try not to swear. The young man's head is right against my chest as I hold the board tight to me. Another firefighter picks up the frame so I don't step on it and sets it on a table by the foot of the stairs. We carry him out the front door and set him on our stretcher, which is just beyond the front steps. I reattach the Ambu bag and hyperventilate him for a moment. His carbon dioxide reading comes back to normal, and the oxygen saturation of his blood is 100 percent.

Before we start to the ambulance, I tell his mother, "Say something to him if you'd like; then we have to go."

"Johnny," she says. She leans down and kisses his face. "I love you, Little Bear. I love you!"

There is no change on the ride to the hospital. His pupils remain fixed. I hang a bag of dopamine from the stretcher IV pole in case his blood pressure drops, but his pressure holds steady. I radio the emergency department: "911 five minutes out with twenty-three-year-old male heroin overdose. Found asystole, got four epis, now in sinus tack with good BP, intubated."

They are ready for us in the resuscitation room. The doctor checks the placement of the breathing tube, and then the respiratory therapist attaches the young man to a ventilator. A nurse draws blood for the lab. The doctor orders cool saline to be run through the patient's two IVs to lower his body temperature. Research has shown that inducing hypothermia can have a protective effect on the brain after a cardiac arrest. He'll be admitted to the intensive care unit (ICU), and the waiting game will begin.

When I turn my run report in, I see his mother and sister sitting outside the room talking with a social worker. Their eyes are red, and they look stunned under the bright hallway lights. A man in a business suit hurries down the hall after being pointed toward them by a nurse. The woman stands, and he takes her in his arms as she cries against his chest. Her wail echoes through the hallway.

A week from today, after the young man's brain shows no signs of electrical activity, the medical staff will take the breathing tube out, and with his family gathered by his side, he will pass away at the age of twenty-three. In their shame, the family will tell friends he died of a congenital heart defect.

The young man was one of 63,632 people to die in America of an accidental overdose in 2016. We thought it was bad then. The numbers would only get worse, with no end in sight.[1]

Hartford, Connecticut, 1995

The year is 1995. A homeless man meets us on the corner of Edgewood and Homestead in the city's north end and leads us into a fire-damaged building. We climb a makeshift ladder to the third floor. We walk down a dark hall and then into a room with broken windows and no furniture. A man sits against the wall with a belt around his bicep and a syringe still in his arm. He is emaciated, probably in his late thirties, with a long, untrimmed beard and boots with holes in the bottoms. By his side is a spoon, a lighter, and a few torn glassine envelopes now devoid of their heroin.

The man is ice cold, and his arms are so stiff with rigor mortis that I can't straighten them. Following protocol, I put a heart monitor on him, run a six-second flatline strip, and then write down the time. From the street below, I can hear pounding rap music from a car driving slowly past. Sirens sound in the distance. We find a wallet in his back pocket with no money in it, just a phone number for a probation officer. We are in walking distance of a community health center and substance use treatment centers, but this man, I reason, obviously loved the needle more than the life he could have had if he'd chosen a straight path. You pick your own destiny, I think.

Many of the overdoses I see in Hartford in my early years as a paramedic are in or around buildings that are abandoned or in disrepair. At the time, there are more than eight hundred condemned buildings in the city. Most of the patients are poor inner-city residents who spend their days committing small robberies or begging for spare change and then scuttling into these vacant buildings to shoot up. Occasionally, we get kids who long ago left the suburban life to come to Hartford for drugs. I don't have sympathy for them. They likely started out as hoods at school, I think, the kind who cut classes and smoke out in the woods, who drop out and let their hair grow long and greasy. They steal from their family and neighbors, become habitual liars, get tattoos, and later get scabs on their arms and faces. They end up begging for change on the street and are found overdosed or dead in their beat-up cars or in the same shooting gallery as this deceased man with drug paraphernalia by their side. I take care of them professionally, but I don't care for them emotionally, certainly not in the same manner I care for an old woman suffering from congestive heart failure, a disabled man with diabetes, or a young woman in a car crash on the highway.

One evening we respond to an overdose in an apartment building. The elevators don't work, and the stairwell smells of urine. A paramedic who arrived in a first-response vehicle does chest compressions on a man in the middle of the floor. Two other men lie slumped on a couch, breathing shallowly. On the table are torn glassine envelopes. The place smells of days-old garbage. "This guy's in arrest," the medic says to us. "Those two need Narcan."

While opioids can bring euphoria to users, opioids also latch onto brain receptors that control breathing. Users' pupils shrink to pinpoints, and their head may drop forward in a prolonged nod as they slip into unconsciousness. As their breathing slows or stops, they become pale and bluish because they no longer have enough oxygen circulating in their blood. If they stop breathing long enough, their heart will stop. This scene in the apartment building shows us users in different stages of overdose.

We draw up two syringes of naloxone, more commonly known as Narcan, the opioid antidote. Naloxone can be administered through an intravenous line, directly into the muscle by injection, or, as later developed, into the nose by nasal spray. Once in the brain, naloxone works by knocking opioids off the brain receptors and allowing the body to breathe again on its own. For this opioid antagonist to work, emergency responders have to get to overdose victims before their heart has stopped. Contrary to myth, naloxone does not revive dead people. We jab the syringe needles in the men's thighs, push the plungers, and then try to shake the men awake. They each arouse before we can get Ambu bags out to assist with their breathing. Their friend isn't so lucky.

I take over doing chest compressions while the other paramedic tries to put a breathing tube in the pulseless man's throat. One of the men we gave Narcan to vomits on the floor while the other sits on the couch and stares at us doing CPR on his friend. He puts his head into his folded arms.

Two women in leather jackets who'd found them shake their heads at the scene. "I fucking told Tommy this would happen if he keeps doing the dope," the brunette says to the policeman interrogating her.

As more help arrives, we secure the man to a long board with three nine-foot straps and begin the extrication. He is in pulseless electrical activity according to the monitor. In this state, the heart still has some electrical juice but isn't able to manage any mechanical function on its own. Only our CPR moves blood to his brain in the faint chance it will keep him alive. It takes four of us to carry him down the stairwell and out to the ambulance. On the way to the hospital, the driver takes a corner fast, and I lose my hand placement on the man's sternum. I stick my hand against his belly to try to keep my balance. My hand decompresses his stomach, which has gathered air from the bagging before the tube was placed. Vomit spews up from his stomach and streams out of his mouth and over his face. It covers his eyes.

"They ought to make this an anti-drug ad," the other medic says with a laugh. An EMT (emergency medical technician) tries to wipe the vomit off while I resume compressions.

At the hospital, the emergency department staff works the overdosed man for another fifteen minutes in the resuscitation room. If he were older, they might not bother. No one in the ED wants to quit on a thirty-year-old, even a heroin user, but the effort seems perfunctory. Everyone in the room knows he is dead. Finally, the doctor, who doesn't look much older than the patient, says, "Enough. 9:17. That's it." The staff quickly exits the room except for the recording nurse. The dead man lies naked on the table, his arms and legs splayed, his skin bluish white, his clothes cut off and strewn on the floor, the plastic breathing tube still sticking out of his mouth. I follow the doctor and watch him go into the room across the hall where one of the other men has been placed.

"Well, your friend's dead," he says angrily. "You keep doing heroin, that's going to be you. If losing a buddy isn't enough to make you stop, I don't know what is. You don't quit, you'll deserve your fate."

The man cries. He is probably twenty-five, but he cries like a nine-year-old.

In 1995, when we talked about the drug problem in Hartford, we were referring to the violence of Hartford's leading gangs, the Latin Kings and Los Solidos, which battled for territory in the Park Street and south end sections of the city, and Twenty Love and the Young Guns, which battled in the north end. In 1994, there were

58 homicides in the city, giving Hartford, a small city with a population of 120,000, one of the highest per capita murder rates in the country at 41.7 per 100,000 people.[1] The Kings wore their colors, black and gold, and the Solidos wore their red and blue as they publicly battled over streets to increase their profits in the drug trade. For a while the killing got so bad that Hartford had to bring in state police to co-patrol the streets with city cops.[2]

One night, after taking a shooting victim with a sucking chest wound to the trauma room at Hartford Hospital, I return to the ambulance and pick up the bloody clothing I had cut off him. In the pockets of his shirt, I find a roll of bills and two small bundles of packets, each held together by a tiny rubber band. They are bundles of heroin. There are ten folded glassine envelopes in each bundle; each is stamped with two six-shooters in red. I take the money and the bloody clothes into the trauma room and lay them on the metal table next to the gurney where the dead man lies. I tell the cop who stands outside the room about the drugs and show him the bags. He hardly seems surprised. "Live by the gun, die by the gun," he says.

The shootings—which occasionally involve innocent bystanders, such as a seven-year-old girl killed by a gang bullet—make headlines, but few pay attention to the drug users, even though the opioid scourge is all around us.[3] The victims of drug use are black, Hispanic, and white, but the deaths never make the news. As a paramedic I often read the obituaries to learn about patients of mine who died. Few of the overdose patients are ever listed. Their life stories are untold. Many are buried in a potter's field without a procession.

One of my partners is an older suburban mom. She lives in a four-bedroom home with an in-ground pool in the backyard and drives a late-model car to work. Sometimes her twenty-six-year-old son meets us at a parking lot where we are posted in the ambulance. (Our company moves ambulances strategically about the city to various locations so as to minimize response times.) My partner always gets out of the ambulance and meets him in the shadows. He is unshaven; his clothes are ragged, and he looks like he hasn't washed in days. She gives him forty dollars and a hushed lecture. "He's a heroin addict," she whispers to me one day. "He's quite troubled. Please don't share. My husband doesn't allow him in our house anymore. God knows where he stays. He's going to end up dead or in jail. I know I shouldn't give him money, but I do. I'm his mother."

You are going to end up dead or in jail. Those words are supposed to make the problem go away. But that is not the way it works. We got it wrong.

Park Street, 2016

It's 2016, and my partner Jerry Sneed drives the ambulance west along Park Street as I ride shotgun. Drug dealing on Park Street is as ubiquitous as the nail salons, bodegas, Spanish restaurants, and boarded-up businesses. Men in hoodies or baseball caps lean against buildings, eyes panning the street. The biggest difference from the 1990s is that the gang colors are gone and shootings are way down. The Kings and the Solidos have learned that attention and violence are bad for profits.[1] The only color that matters is green. Driving slowly by in the ambulance, we watch the transactions. Some users walk down an alley behind the Bean Pot Restaurant to make the deal in the rear parking lot, while others buy their drugs in the open. The dealers give a quick handshake, the small folded heroin envelopes briefly visible in their palms. Some lean into a car to chat and make an exchange.

One morning we watch black unmarked SUVs screech to the curb and vested undercover agents charge into the same alley with guns drawn. Dealers and users are turned around, thrown up against the alley wall, searched, and cuffed. They are led out to a paddy wagon that takes those ensnared away, but the next day, dealers are back at it. Take out a dealer or shut down a block, it doesn't matter; there is always someone else ready to sell.

Heroin in Hartford, along with most of the East Coast, is sold primarily in a powdered form. A 0.1 g bag of heroin doesn't contain enough powder to cover the bowl of a spoon but more than enough to kill an opioid-naïve person—someone who's never tried the drug. A single bag goes for $4 on the city streets. The cost is $30 for a bundle of ten, $125 for a brick of fifty, or $200 for a stack of one hundred bags. The farther you get from the city, the higher the price. If you are from the suburbs and are tired of paying a premium to your local dealer, you do what he likely does: head in to Hartford. If you have never been there before, just walk down Park Street or drive your car slowly down the avenue, and the dealers will find you. Business is booming. They hawk their brands, which are stamped or printed on the bags: Black Jack, Easy Money, Skull and Bones, Diesel, Scorpion, The Truth, Killing Time. They've got what you need, plus a beeper number for your next trip into the city.

We watch the users, wearing backpacks and often walking in pairs. Their purchases made, they head west, crossing Park Terrace toward Pope Park. Some descend into the thick underbrush. Their prior visits have carved out little warrens hidden beneath the high shrubbery, circles of packed earth where, amid discarded trash and the stink of urine, they sit on milk crates or an old tire and shoot up out of sight of traffic. Others head deeper into Pope Park, seventy acres of public athletic fields, benches, giant trees, and a pavilion by a pond. The pavilion is a popular place for users, as they can sit on the hard floor with their back against a brick wall and use without interference. Across the street to the north is 1200 Park, a shopping plaza with a laundromat, a cut-rate grocery store, two dollar stores, a liquor store, an auto parts store, a furniture store, two clothing shops, a dental office, and cell phone store in one long building; and in a smaller building, across the spacious parking lot, stands a Subway restaurant, a nail studio, and another cell phone store. To the west is the elevated Interstate 84, underneath which homeless people often set up camps, just out of sight from the parking lot on property owned by Amtrak. Users frequently buy their drugs east on Park and then drive to the Plaza, where they shoot up in their cars or use the restrooms in the laundromat or at the Subway.

That's where we're headed now. Jerry hits the lights on as he acknowledges the call on the radio. "1200 Park. Subway. Priority one. Man unconscious in the restroom."

A stocky bearded man in his thirties sits on the toilet, his pants down around his legs. His head is against the wall; his mouth is open, but he is not breathing. His skin is cyanotic (blue). His pupils are pinpoint. He is warm and has a pounding carotid pulse in his neck. I shake him hard. He does not respond to stimulation. While Jerry gets out the Ambu bag, I take out the Narcan and inject 1.2 milligrams into his bare thigh. I am getting ready to put a hard-plastic oral airway in his mouth to keep his tongue from blocking his breathing passageway, when suddenly he wakes and looks up with a start to see me standing over him holding the oral airway, my partner with the Ambu bag, and three firefighters.

"You're in a public bathroom," I say. "You overdosed. We just gave you Narcan."

"Overdosed? I didn't overdose."

"You weren't breathing. We gave you Narcan."

He swears. "I'm fine. You all can leave."

"You did heroin."

"Heroin? I don't know what you are talking about." He looks away from me quickly, his eyes darting about the room, eyelids blinking.

"Quit lying," a firefighter says. "We just saved your life. You should be grateful."

"Stand up and put your pants on," Jerry says quietly.

"What are you talking about?"

"You are sitting on a toilet. Your pants are around your ankles. Pull your pants up. The bathroom door's wide open."

The man stands with our help, and we get his pants up. He glances furtively toward the open bathroom door. If there were not so many people in the bathroom, I think he might try to bolt.

"You recognize these?" Jerry shows him two empty heroin bags he'd found by the sink; the bags bear the words "Black Jack" and a printed picture of two playing cards—the ace of hearts and the king of spades.

"Those aren't mine."

"How about this syringe?" Jerry holds up an orange-capped 1 cc syringe.

"No, I told you I don't do drugs."

"Okay," I say. "We are taking you to the hospital."

His forehead is beaded with sweat. I hand him a vomit bag, which he proceeds to fill with vomit on the way to the hospital. The naloxone, while restoring his breathing, has put him into full-scale withdrawal. Instead of the bliss he sought, his muscles are aching, he is sweating from every pore, and his stomach is cramping. He vomits again.

At the emergency department, I give my report to Nancy, the ED nurse at the patient's bedside. She is in her late twenties, an otherwise attractive young woman except for the clear annoyance on her face as she looks at him like he is there only to cause her trouble. The ED is crowded with beds already overflowing in the hallways.

"He says he didn't do drugs," I tell her, "but he came around with 1.2 of Narcan."

"I don't do drugs," he tells her, in between retches.

"Yeah, and this is the Plaza Hotel," she responds.

An hour later, we get a call for an unconscious person in a car. The car is in the parking lot of a bodega on Broad Street, which is a major road that leads directly from Park Street to Interstate 84.

Customers buy drugs on Park Street and then find a place to shoot up before they go back to the suburbs—at least those who can't wait to get back to their town to use.

Two firefighters bang on the door of the Toyota. The man inside looks at them but seems to be in a stupor. "Open the door! Open the door!" the firefighters yell. He doesn't move. They use a bar to pop the lock.

Jerry opens the door. "You're not in trouble; we just need to check you out," he says.

A young man in a bright white t-shirt with a thin-cut mohawk is finally persuaded to step out, but then he makes a sudden move back inside the car to grab something—a syringe. Jerry bear-hugs him before he can fully grasp it. There is a short wrestling match and shouting. A police officer throws the man up against the car. I retrieve the 1 cc syringe that the man had dropped on the floorboard; 0.5 cubic centimeters of brownish water with a ribbon of blood is left in the syringe barrel. The needle is bent. I dispose of it in our ambulance's sharps box while Jerry gets the man on the stretcher. The man is trembling and very sweaty. Along the length of each of his forearms is a colorful dragon tattoo. With the police officer, I do a quick check in the car for additional information. We find ten empty heroin bags in the console. A bundle. It's a new brand: OMG, or "Oh My God," with stars on it.

In the ambulance, the man is tachycardic: his heart rate races at 140 beats a minute. He says he has not used in four days. His pupils are pinpoint. Sweat beads on his forehead. He bleeds slightly from a vein in his hand. I am guessing he nodded off halfway through his hit with the syringe still in his hand vein. He didn't inject enough to get rid of the sickness. He won't get Narcan from us, even though he nods off at times during the ride. I give him fluid through an IV and Zofran, an anti-nausea medicine.

"I hurt my shoulder lifting weights," he tells me when I ask how he got started. "My doctor gave me Percocets. I got hooked."

He has been to rehab several times. He tells me he called a beeper number and then met his contact by the bakery on Park. "Thank you for helping me," he says. "I want to get back into rehab. I will never do drugs again."

He shakes our hands at the hospital once we help him to his ED room. I write on a piece of paper the address where his car is parked and hand it to him. Jerry gets him a pillow for his head.

"Again?" Nancy says. "What? The hospital across town is closed?"

"We like seeing you," Jerry says. "How's our guy from before?"

"Oh, lovely man," she says with disdain. "He left AMA after stealing half a tray of my IV supplies." (By AMA, she means he left against medical advice.)

Later that afternoon we are driving down Park Street. I see the young man with a distinctive mohawk in a white t-shirt with dragon tattoos on his forearms standing in a doorway of a boarded-up store, talking on a cell phone. He puts the cell phone in his pocket and then walks into the bakery next door.

The sad fact is that neither Jerry nor I are surprised by this. When heroin users are in withdrawal and you don't find a way to get them directly into treatment, they are going to make a beeline back to Park Street.

Antipathy

Doctors, nurses, paramedics, EMTs, cops, and firefighters can all be rough-edged toward drug users. Drug users often present health care providers with the difficult situation of dealing with patients who are uncooperative, untruthful, and even combative. They may present this way because they are sick and believe that we, as health care providers, aren't going to provide them with what they need—pain medicine to stave off withdrawal. Furthermore, they may suspect we will stigmatize them as scum and deadbeats because they are addicted to drugs. In many cases, their fears are justified. Some health care providers feel disgust toward drug users, believing they have brought their situation on themselves through their own character flaws; others are hard with users as a front to block the emotions that come from the daily onslaught of people in need of help whom they deal with in their jobs. The term for this is *compassion fatigue*. It is also known as moral injury.[1]

In paramedic school in 1992, an instructor stands in front of our class and tells us how, if ever there's a triage nurse at a hospital we don't like or who has been disrespectful to us, he knows a great way to get back at her: "Get an IV, draw up 2 milligrams of naloxone, place the needle in the IV port, and then just as you come through the ED doors, push the Narcan hard and fast. Your patient will sit bolt upright, and if your timing is right, they'll unleash a spray of vomit right at the triage nurse."

He tells us this trick with bravado. The class laughs nervously, uncertain whether we might actually find ourselves doing this someday—weaponizing a heroin user to retaliate against a battle-axe nurse who shows us insufficient respect. What kind of world are we about to enter?

When I graduate from medic school in 1993, only paramedics can carry and administer naloxone in the field. Paramedics are advanced providers who undergo usually about two additional years of school beyond the typical 120 hours of training an EMT receives. Initially, naloxone is given only intravenously, with an injection through an intravenous line, or intramuscularly, with a needle shot directly into a muscle, usually the thigh or upper arm. Many years later, a new delivery method is popularized: intranasal. In this method an atomizer is attached to the syringe and inserted into a patient's nostril. When you push the syringe plunger briskly, the fluid is forced through the atomizer and turned into a fine mist. The aerosolized particles are small enough to penetrate the blood-brain barrier and provide an active response. One milligram in each nostril usually does the trick. This method enables people without advanced medical training to administer the drug easily. As the opioid epidemic grows worse, more and more states allow EMTs, first responders, and laypeople to carry and administer naloxone.

I arrive on the scene of a car accident. The police officer directing traffic says to me, "You're going to need your Narcan." I find the patient slumped over the steering wheel, not breathing. I give him naloxone, and we breathe for him until he wakes with a jolt. But all that time, I am thinking how much quicker and easier it would have been for the police officer to have squirted some naloxone up the man's nose when he first arrived, if only the law had allowed him to carry it. Fortunately, Connecticut later becomes one of the states permitting first responders to carry the drug, and in early 2017, the Hartford police are equipped with this lifesaving medicine, along with members of the fire department, who started carrying it a year earlier. Nationally, most first responders embrace the additional responsibility of carrying naloxone, while others, who have little interest in providing aid to drug users, resist.

Early in 2016, a firefighter in Weymouth, Massachusetts, posts on Facebook, "Narcan is the worst drug ever created, let the [expletive] bags die. . . . I for one get no extra money for giving Narcan and these losers are out of the hospital and using again in hours, you use—you should lose." The chief of the fire department suspends him for ninety days without pay and states, "The comments posted do not reflect the philosophy or values we hold as a fire department or town."[2]

The story makes national news. Although the fire chief issues the statement disavowing the man's post, the man, who later apologizes for his comments, is clearly not alone in his views. On many online discussion boards, emergency personnel echo his anti-Narcan and anti-drug-user sentiments, while other emergency medical services (EMS) personnel join in to condemn users.[3] A poster writes, "Instead of trumpeting the number of saves they should be keeping track of the number of repeats." Another writes, "Where do you want your ambulance to go? An elderly person with CHF, a factory worker bleeding out from an industrial accident, a child [having] difficulty breathing, or a repeat OD that will yell at you afterwards because he'll have to score again to regain his high?" Another commenter scolds them: "Go to the job and do it to the best of your ability. We're not there to judge and what is happening to some of these folks, can happen to anyone."[4]

In 2018, a state police dispatcher in Brockton, Massachusetts, is put on administrative leave for posting on Facebook that, instead of reviving a pregnant woman with naloxone, she should have been "left to rot." The dispatcher went on: "Phuck that disease bullshit 'disease' crap. Selfish piece of shit!"[5] Again, the EMS message boards display a surprising amount of sympathy for this dispatcher and her viewpoint.

A Hartford police officer is reassigned while being investigated for posting a photo on Facebook of the intersection of Park and Hudson Streets and commenting, "Every [expletive] parasite in the city passes through this [expletive] intersection at least once a day! It's 10 AM and it's been half a dozen hookers, several dozen junkies, lost suburbanites looking for Heroin. . . . Someone do me a solid and call in an air strike!"[6]

Just this past year, on my own company's employees-only Facebook page, an EMT posts a link to a YouTube video of an opioid user standing on a street corner, clearly on the nod, his head bent forward, asleep on his feet. Another man sneaks up on him. He hauls back and hits the heroin user hard across the face. The victim grabs his head and starts running blindly down the street as if he has just been attacked by invisible aliens. The assailant meanwhile has escaped to the other side of the street.[7] The clip captioned "The Fastest Way to Sober Up Heroin Addicts" gets a few almost instantaneous laugh-out-loud comments before it is taken down by a board administrator for being inappropriate.

Imagine a paramedic posting a video of a stranger stomping on an old woman lying on the ground with a hip fracture. No EMS provider or any health care provider would ever think of making such a post. But when it comes to drug use, it's open season for bashing the users. The reasons are a lack of understanding about substance use and, sadly at times, a lack of empathy.

Richard K. Jones, the sheriff of Butler County, Ohio, won't permit his deputies to carry naloxone. In an interview with the

Washington Post, he declares, "We don't do the shots for bee stings, we don't inject diabetic people with insulin. When does it stop? . . . I'm not the one that decides if people live or die. They decide that when they stick that needle in their arm."[8]

In the same county in Ohio, council member Dan Picard proposes a three-strikes-you're-out policy for drug users. The county would issue a summons to anyone overdosing twice and require them to do community service. Their name would go in a database after a second conviction. "We'll have that list and when we get a call, the dispatcher will ask who is the person who has overdosed," Picard says to the *Washington Post*. "And if it's someone who has already been provided services twice, we'll advise them that we're not going to provide further services—and we will not send out an ambulance."[9]

Again, imagine an ambulance not responding to a woman in her third car accident or a cigarette smoker with chronic obstructive pulmonary disease calling for the third time because of shortness of breath or a man with coronary artery disease and a liking for bacon having a third heart attack. Imagine one human being standing over another human being who is dying and doing nothing even though that person holds the medicine capable of reviving the one who's dying.

Fire Captain Gary LeBlanc of Waterbury, Connecticut, is in a meeting about whether the firefighters should start carrying naloxone when one of his fellow firefighters says, "We ought to just let these scumbags die." LeBlanc, who has never spoken of his family situation to his fellow firefighters before, turns to his brother firefighter and says, "So you want my son Jeremy to die, huh?" The man immediately backs down.

LeBlanc then embarks on a campaign to tell EMS groups about the crisis that his family is enduring. At an event I attend, he brings his son with him, and the two tell the story of a young man who grew up loved and provided for by his family, who suffered undiagnosed anxiety and depression. When he is hurt in an accident and given oxycodone, he feels like the drug fills a hole he didn't know he had. He follows the same path that many others have tumbled down: his prescription runs out, so he starts buying pills, ends up injecting the cheaper and stronger heroin, and becomes homeless. With the love of his family behind him, he makes it through rehab several times and is now working toward a degree as a counselor for other users. He says he still thinks about using every day. The two receive a standing ovation for their talk. Yet by the end of the symposium, some audience members who had applauded the LeBlancs' talk fall back into remarking about how annoying it is to have to give someone Narcan several times in the same day and questioning whether trading heroin for methadone or Suboxone, two drugs often prescribed to users to break them of their heroin habit, is just trading one addiction for another. I used to feel that way until I was educated about the utility of these drugs. Yes, it is trading one opioid for another, but an addiction to heroin or fentanyl is much more likely to kill someone or to destroy families, jobs, and lives, while patients who receive methadone or Suboxone under a doctor's order are much more likely to have jobs where they pay taxes, have intact families, and, most important, are far less likely to die of overdose.

Why do so many have so much antipathy toward drug users? If you don't understand the science behind addiction, and if you believe (as I used to) that addiction is a character flaw and not a disease, it is easy to believe the stereotype and point the finger at the user.

"Don't lie to us," an EMT says to a disheveled man whom he finds unresponsive in the park bushes. "What were you doing down here? Of course, you were using drugs! Look at your track-marked arms. We gave you Narcan. We saved your life! You ought to be thanking us, instead of lying to us. Now get on the stretcher! You're going to the hospital. It's that or the PD is going to take you to the lockup. Come on, let's go. We don't have all day. There's other people in the city who truly need ambulances."

If providers cannot treat patients decently, I believe they should move into work that doesn't involve direct patient contact. That doesn't mean they are bad people. Emergency medical work is traumatizing. It can rob some providers' hearts of kindness. In my mind, someone who loses his compassion is no different from someone who has ruptured a disc in his back from traumatic lifting. They are both broken. As I wouldn't want someone with a blown-out back carrying a patient down a steep set of stairs, I don't want someone with a blown-out compassion center treating someone who has just been resuscitated from a heroin overdose.

Today, I am quite pious about the need to treat users as patients—as victims of a horrible disease who need our compassion and best care efforts—but I have a confession of my own to make.

I wrote a book, published in 1998, called *Paramedic: On the Front Lines of Medicine*, about my first year as a paramedic. I picked up the book the other day, after not having looked at it in years, to see how I characterized any heroin overdoses I wrote about. In a chapter about struggling with burnout—which is not uncommon for a new paramedic trying to understand the fatigue and emotions of responding day after day to constant 911 calls, many of them for people who don't seem to care for themselves or appreciate what you are trying to do for them—I described finding a man unresponsive from a heroin overdose, revving him with enough Narcan to restore his breathing, and then having to carry him down three steep, narrow flights of stairs.

Here is a portion of what I wrote:

> The cop stands behind me holding my belt to keep me from tumbling backward. The guy's feet are hitting my knees. Both Glenn and I are irritable. The small of my back feels like it's going to explode. I look at the guy we are carrying with revulsion. I have done countless

overdoses and drunks and though I have never said it to a patient of mine, I want to say, "Scumbag." I think I could have slammed a heavy dose right into his veins without even bothering to do an IV, "hotwiring" him, bringing him from deep heroin bliss to puking nausea. If he got violent, the cop could have smacked him with his billy club. I think I should have at least given him enough so he could stand, however wobbly, and we could have dragged him along, step by step, so we wouldn't be carrying him in this heat, with our backs threatening to explode, and the two of us yelling at each other to go slow, or speed up, or lift better. I look at him and think, Scumbag.[10]

Empathy

My recognition that drug users might be more than just scum was gradual, but one call stands out clearly in my recollection.

At the scene is a car driven into a pole in front of the gas station at Sisson and Park. We are told that it is a possible drug overdose. There is minor damage to the front end of the Ford, but its driver, a young woman in a white tank top with long-stem rose tattoos down both of her forearms, is slumped over the steering wheel. She is blue and not breathing, but she has a pounding carotid pulse. We pull her out of the car and onto our stretcher. A syringe is on the seat next to her, along with several torn glassine envelopes stamped "Sweet Heart" in red ink. Her pupils are pinpoint. While my partner breathes for her with an Ambu bag, I squirt 2 milligrams of naloxone up her nose.

She comes around in the back of the ambulance. She seems familiar to me with her freckles. I may have had her as a patient in the past. "I was doing so good," she says, sadly. "I got out of rehab three weeks ago. I've been clean. I just slipped up."

I hear this all the time. *I just slipped up. I've been clean.* At first, I don't believe it. I think people are just making excuses. But that is before I learn about developing tolerance to a drug. Tolerance means either you have to use more opioid to get the same effect or you get less of an effect when using the same amount.[1] When you take opioids for a while, your body gets used to them, and you need to take more to maintain the same effect. Many people on prescription pain meds go back to their doctor for stronger prescriptions. Heroin users go from needing two bags a day to shooting ten bags at a time just to keep from going into withdrawal. When they stop using for a while, they no longer need as much. People getting out of jail, getting out of rehab, or falling off the wagon after a period of abstinence have lost their tolerance. If they take their former usual amount of heroin or number of pills, they can easily overdose, as it is now too much for their system. These people are the ones who are most at risk for a fatal overdose.

"Besides substance abuse," I ask, "do you have any other medical problems?"

"I broke my back cheerleading," she says.

I remember her now in her red uniform, the scared look in her eyes as everyone gathered around her where she had fallen.

"They dropped you?" I say. She nods. I mention the name of the town.

"That was me," she says.

Years ago we put a cervical collar on her neck and lifted her carefully on a backboard. We drove slowly to the hospital, taking care not to hit the potholes. Her father in the front seat kept asking how she was doing, which was quite fine, as I had given her IV morphine that made all her worries go away.

"Do you mind if I ask how you ended up like this?"

"A heroin user?"

"I didn't mean it like that," I said, catching the combination of defensiveness and defiance in her tone. "I'm curious if you want to tell me."

And so she does. "I had surgery and had to miss a lot of school," she says. "Life wasn't great. I was on Percocets for a year, and then my doctor told me I didn't need them anymore. I did."

She tells me she bought pills from a high school classmate to fight off the sickness of withdrawal. When she had trouble affording the pills, the same guy introduced her to heroin. It looked like powdered sugar. All she had to do was snort it. No tying a belt around her bicep and sticking a needle into her arm. Just raise it to your nose and inhale. It was stronger and cheaper than the pills. But then her tolerance grew, and it wasn't long before she tied a USB cord around her arm and hit her first vein. It was the only way she could get relief.

"I used to be a normal girl," she says.

The more I hear users say that to me, the more I begin to understand they are speaking the truth. I wonder what her life would have been like if she could return to that moment when she was flying through the air before the football crowd on a beautiful October evening, the sun setting on the orange and red New England hills. She is in her tight spiral, a picture-perfect moment. All her life is ahead of her. What if her squad caught her this time when she came down? The crowd would have roared. She would have smiled and done a cartwheel. Her life could have followed a completely different trajectory—high school dances, prom queen, college, an engagement ring, a house with a white picket fence, kids playing in the yard, and perhaps a career. Instead, those dreams now disappear into a hole in her arm.

"How did you get involved with opioids in the first place?" I start asking my patients. Within a short time their answers make the horror of the epidemic come alive to me and make me completely change the views I hold. No one tells me, "I just decided to become a heroin addict." Instead, this is what I hear: "I got into a car crash and broke my back." "I tore up my knee skiing." "I got shot as a fourteen-year-old standing on a street corner." "I got hit by a car." "I had a stomach tumor." I call up to my partner Jerry, who is driving us to the hospital each time a patient reveals her opioid origin story. Each is a eureka moment for me. "Car accident!" I call to Jerry. "Football injury!" "Fell off a roof!" Each patient proves the new thesis. Many people's addiction starts with an injury, a random event. They are prescribed pain meds by their doctor. The spiral begins.

We find a man lying underneath the hedges of a yard on Collins Street just a block from Saint Francis Hospital. A construction crew working on a nearby roof spotted him and called 911. He rouses with stimulation, and after he gets to his feet, he tells us he has been sleeping there. He seems unsteady. He is a thin, unshaven man in his late thirties with pinpoint pupils. His clothes are dirty. He wears tattered boots and a green work jacket. He admits he has come to the city looking for pills. He says he bought some yesterday and spent the night in the bushes. He has no pills left and no money. I ask him where he lives, and he says he is now homeless. He hurt his back in a work accident and got addicted to pain pills. That addiction has cost him his family, his business, and his home in the suburbs. "I have nowhere to go," he says. Maybe it is the coat that so clearly spells out his decline, with "Dan's Tree Service" patched on the right breast and "Dan" patched on the left, which is all he has left of a life that once made him proud.

I wonder what his life would have been like if he hadn't gotten hurt. Maybe today he would be at his daughter's school piano recital. He gets there in the nick of time. His daughter smiles in relief before striking the piano keys, as he settles in next to his pretty, young wife, who squeezes his hand, grateful he has made it. She knows that he rises early every morning, puts on his working clothes, and provides for them.

"Come on, we'll take you to the hospital," I say now. "You can sleep there for a little bit and get something to eat."

I am noticing more and more patients like him—lost souls, displaced from their lives, ending up on Hartford's streets. What happened to them? When did their lives come apart? An EMT tells me of getting a text from a favorite high school teacher who asks to borrow money. She thinks it so odd and does not answer. He must have texted her by mistake. A month later, she picks him up overdosed on Park Street and finds a pawn ticket for a car in his wallet. A young paramedic I am training tells me of encountering an overdose victim, a fellow student from her training class who had dropped out and disappeared after the first semester. She hurt her back lifting a patient, got hooked on pain pills, and lost control. She just got out of recovery and had been doing well until she slipped up again.

I used to think that being a great paramedic came from having medical skills: the ability to get an IV in a critical patient with poor veins, to insert a tracheal tube in an unconscious patient, or to recognize a lethal cardiac rhythm and shock it before the patient stops breathing. In time I begin to see that a paramedic's job is about more than just providing the medicine; it is about listening to patients, observing, trying to understand their lives, and treating them with decency.

Empathy is the ability to see life through another's eyes. To thrive long term in the emergency medicine field, you have to have it. The turnover rate in EMS is extremely high. Many realize it is not for them, and they leave. Others who may come to a similar understanding, unfortunately, get stuck in the field. They start in EMS at a young age and make good money (thanks to near-unlimited overtime). Later on they find themselves without a college degree and no other line of work where they can make the same income. As they grow older, they find it harder and harder to endure the endless hours and the toll of the job on their body.

Years of treating, carrying, and dealing with people who don't always appreciate it can turn some hearts bitter, which affects the responder's life, family, and health. Sadly, a number of people I have worked with over the years ended up taking their own life. Some simply drank themselves to death or accidentally overdosed on drugs after having become addicted to painkillers they started taking for a job-related injury; others ended their lives violently. A recent study found suicide rates high among first responders: 6.6 percent had attempted suicide, and 37 percent had contemplated it. According to the Centers for Disease Control and Prevention, this suicide attempt rate was thirteen times the national average, while the contemplation rate was ten times higher than in the general population.[2] How does this affect first responders? It can make them build outer walls of toughness through which they show no weakness or compassion. It can give them a hard edge that hampers their ability to show empathy for others.

I have my periods of darkness on the job, but I have more years of light. I always enjoy the array of people I take care of, and the more I learn about my patients, the more I come to understand the circumstances of their lives. It does not take long, with all the substance use calls I respond to, for me to see that these people aren't scumbags. They aren't bad people; many have just had bad fortune. None of these people willingly chose the life they are leading.

On one call I stand over another overdose victim found in the bushes off Park Terrace, his life come to an end, slumped face forward in a thicket, his body resting on a mat of old heroin bags, empty saline vials, and syringe caps. In his worn wallet, devoid of cash, there are faded and crumpled school pictures of two young children. Before he took his final shot, had he been offered to trade his life now for the life he had then, I don't think he would have hesitated a moment to go back in time. Sadly, people who have become addicted to opioids cannot escape their condition by clicking their heels and wishing they were home.

Addiction

A call comes over the radio: "911. Priority one. Signal seventeen in Hartford, unresponsive in a car. Capitol and Broad at the gas station."

"Sounds like another OD," Jerry says, flicking our red lights on. "No doubt."

We are just three blocks away and arrive before police or firefighters. A woman, cell phone in hand, stands in front of the convenience mart and points without smiling to a gray SUV parked in one of the side spaces. The driver is slumped over the wheel. The vehicle is locked, but the window is down enough for me to reach in and pop the button. I open the door and gently shake the driver, a pale, thin woman in her thirties wearing a tank top and yoga pants. No response. When I shake her again, harder this time, she looks up at me vacantly. Drool comes from her mouth. In the back seat are two children, who, I'm guessing, are three and five years old. They are not smiling. I shake her again. She focuses on me. "Are you diabetic?" I ask.

"No." She looks around in a sudden panic. She sees her children. "Oh, Christ," she says. She looks out the window and sees that she is at a gas station. "I must have. I must have fallen asleep."

Her pupils are pinpoint—my clear suspicion is opioid use. I look on the floor of the car for any envelopes or paraphernalia. "You need to tell me what's going on here so I can help you."

"Nothing."

I look at the five-year-old. She stares back at me with the eyes of someone of far more years. Whatever she knows, she's not going to tell me.

"I just fell asleep," the mother says. "I'm tired."

"We need to take you to the hospital."

"No, no. I'm fine."

I hear an approaching siren. "The police are coming," I say, "and they are not going to let you drive with your kids in the car."

"No, no really."

"Do you have someone you can call to come get them?"

"My husband. He's at work. I don't want to bother him. I'm fine, really, I'm fine. I was just tired. I didn't sleep well last night."

"You need to call him. They are not going to let you drive."

She gets her cell phone out and calls. "Honey," she says. "I fell asleep in the car at a gas station. The kids are all right." I can hear him yelling at her.

"Where am I?" she asks me.

"Broad Street, near Capitol," I say. She tells him. He yells some more.

When she finally hangs up, she says, "He's coming."

"I have to ask," I say, "what did you take?"

"I didn't get any sleep last night. I have chronic pain."

"You can't be driving like this with your kids in the car."

"I know," she says.

A police officer arrives, and I explain what I have seen: "She was passed out at the wheel. Her husband is coming to get the kids. Her pupils are pinpoint. She says she didn't sleep well last night."

The officer barks at her. "What did you take?"

The woman just cries.

The officer shakes his head and takes her license number and runs her plates. In another part of town, he might have a different reaction, but where we are is a common rest stop for users. People come into the city to buy drugs on Park Street. They drive back to the highway and stop at this service station. If they are drug sick, they may get a quick fix in what they think is an inconspicuous place before getting back on the highway. Sometimes, however, they wake up to find themselves surrounded by people in uniform.

Jerry points to the ground outside the car window. Two torn bags of heroin. Stamped on them in black ink are the words "The Purge." They could be from her, or they could be from anyone else who has parked here since the manager last swept the lot. He sweeps often.

"Where's your husband coming from?" I ask the woman.

"He's just a few minutes away."

The woman starts to nod off. I give her another shake. She awakens.

A pickup truck pulls into the gas station, and a tall broad-shouldered man with a crew cut steps out. He is wearing a bulletproof vest under his sweatshirt. He strides right to the car and ignores my effort to make eye contact before I tell him what is going on.

"Are you okay?" he says to the children. The three-year-old starts crying.

"I'm sorry," the wife says.

"This is the last fucking time," he says to her. He glares at her as I explain what I saw. He nods and says, "I'll take the kids."

I watch him secure them safely in the back seat of his pickup. My partner and I get the woman on our stretcher. Her husband talks with the cop. They appear to know each other. They lock her car up. The man says he'll come back for it. We tell him we are taking her to Saint Francis Hospital. He doesn't say goodbye.

On the way to the hospital, she sobs. "He's going to divorce me and take my children," she says. She admits to me that she uses pain pills and has a problem.

"How did you get started with pain pills?"

"I had two caesarians," she says. "I don't tolerate pain well. My doctor is trying to taper me off the pills, but it isn't working."

"Did you use heroin this morning?"

"No," she says.

"What were you doing in Hartford?"

She looks down.

"You getting some help is going to be the best thing for your family."

"I know," she says. "I was doing so good."

Too many times of late in the news are accounts and graphic photos of a parent found overdosed in a car with children in the back seat or an infant found at home suckling a mother who still has a syringe in her arm. An Ohio police officer takes pictures from both sides of a car with a mother and father overdosed in the front seat while their four-year-old son looks on from the back. In the photos, the father sits with his head tilted back, his mouth open. His wife is slumped in the passenger seat, also out cold, her mouth open. The police post the images on Facebook with a message: "We feel it necessary to show the other side of this horrible drug. We feel we need to be a voice for the children caught up in this horrible mess. This child can't speak for himself but we are hopeful his story can convince another user to think twice about injecting this poison while having a child in their custody." The police department receives much criticism for posting the photos. The department responds, "We are well aware some may be offended by these images and for that we are truly sorry. But it is time that the non-drug using public sees what we are dealing with on a daily basis."[1]

The police department's disregard for the family's privacy is appalling. Imagine having to live in a community as the publicly shamed parents who overdosed in front of their child or as the publicly identified child neglected by his parents. I can only believe that the police official who made the decision to publish the photos never received training in addiction or the consequences of stigma, which I am only beginning to understand fully myself. (In Hartford, and in most cities and towns in Connecticut, police officers now carry naloxone, with which they revive overdosed persons instead of taking pictures of them while waiting for the paramedics to arrive and administer the lifesaving drug.)

The behavior we see in emergency services is not normal. How is it possible that some people love getting high more than they love their own children? It is hard to comprehend for those of us who consider taking care of children to be a defining part of life. To understand what is happening, we have to look at the science of addiction. I have been reading as much as I can about it to make sense of this epidemic.

The American Psychiatric Association defines addiction as "a complex condition, a brain disease that is manifested by compulsive substance use despite harmful consequence."[2] The Society of Addiction Medicine says addiction "is characterized by [an] inability to consistently abstain, impairment in behavioral control, craving, diminished recognition of significant problems with one's behaviors and interpersonal relationships, and a dysfunctional emotional response."[3]

I read an article in the *New York Times* about opioid users who were shown pictures of cute babies while having their brains scanned.[4] The users' brains failed to light up in the area of the brain associated with emotional rewards, while the brains of healthy volunteers lit up as expected. When the users were given an opioid blocker called naltrexone, their response to the babies' pictures improved. Comments on the newspaper's website mock the study for showing the obvious—opioid addicts are not good parents—but they miss the point. The study shows that the brains of opioid users are diseased and no longer functioning properly, explaining why they may not be good parents.

On the website of the National Institute on Drug Abuse, there is a brain scan of a drug user along with one from a healthy person.[5] You can see the user's disease as clearly as a disease in someone with a kidney tumor, bad lungs, or a brain bleed. The scientific truth is that users have a disease that impairs their brain functioning. I imagine that to expect them to act rationally is akin to expecting someone with chronic obstructive lung disease to run a marathon or someone with congestive heart failure to climb Mount Everest. I understand now that people who shoot up in front of their kids are not intrinsically horrible people; what they are is damaged.

At seminars I attend, I hear substance abuse physicians describe the explosion of pleasure in our brain when we have sex or eat delicious food. The pleasure is caused by our brain releasing dopamine, a feel-good chemical. Physicians use the analogy of fireworks. Let's say five fireworks of dopamine go off when we have sex or eat our favorite pizza. Later, when we think about having sex or eating, more fireworks go off. These activities are associated with pleasure. Eating and having sex are keys to our survival as human beings, so our brain is programmed to reward these acts. It drives us toward them. If we don't eat and don't have sex, then we won't survive as a species. That's why our brain rewards us with fireworks when we partake in them and even rewards us when we think about partaking. We are also programmed to care for our young. We look at a cute baby and feel warm and protective toward it. That positive response is programmed in us to ensure a future for humans on earth.

Now let's say we try heroin for the first time. Instead of five fireworks going off in our brain, fifty fireworks of dopamine go off. For those who are more genetically disposed to the drug, it may be a hundred fireworks. Not every brain can handle such an explosion. The pleasure center (in the basal ganglia) is suddenly overwhelmed with a hundred-year flood of dopamine. After that initial explosion, another part of the brain (the extended amygdala) notices that the wondrous feeling is subsiding, and then a third part of the brain (the prefrontal cortex) starts thinking about getting some more heroin. The cycle has begun. Unfortunately, each time a person does heroin, the brain becomes more accustomed to it, the number of fireworks is fewer, and the brain fixates harder on obtaining more. Only more heroin can produce that dopamine rush that fuels the brain's reward system. The brain has become rewired. Instead of sex and food and protecting babies being the key to survival, heroin hijacks the brain and reorders priorities: heroin is the key. Sex and food and protecting babies no longer trigger a dopamine response significant enough to bring pleasure. The brain believes all that matters to its survival is getting more heroin.[6]

I learn two sad facts.

One, the younger someone is when exposed to opioids, the more likely that person is to suffer long-term addiction because young people's brains are not fully formed. The bypass pathway is more easily rewired because the brain is still malleable. Research published in *Pediatrics* in November 2015 found that, when prescribed an opioid before their senior year in high school, people with no drug use history and who strongly disapprove of others smoking marijuana have a 33 percent greater risk of engaging in harmful opioid use later in life than those who had no opioid prescription.[7]

Two, the great dopamine explosion that a user first feels may never occur again with the same intensity. With each use, the level of dopamine recedes, as does the ability to produce dopamine for the things that used to cause pleasure. When users continue using regularly, they will reach a point when they must get high simply to keep from feeling sick. The phrase "chasing the dragon" can mean smoking heroin, but it can also mean chasing that first glorious high and never finding it again.[8] The drug that once brought unbelievable euphoria is now desperately needed as medicine to hold sickness at bay.

On a cold, rainy day, I find a young man huddled in the trees and trying to inject himself. I hold my hands up in a gesture of peace. His arms are bleeding in multiple places. He holds a loaded syringe in his hands. He can't find a vein. I wish I could help him, but I can't. Instead, I give him a few dollars to get a cup of coffee. He tells me he started using opioids as a fourteen-year-old who was sent to the pharmacy each week to pick up his cancer-ridden mother's pain pills. She shared those pills with him whenever he had a headache or trouble sleeping. By eighteen he was using heroin. "I've dived head first into all sorts of drugs, but you can escape them all except heroin," he says. "Heroin grabs you by the ankles when you try to get away, and it pulls you back in. It makes you suffer when you try to leave it, and it never loves you again like it once did."

One time we are flagged down by passersby and pointed to a car stopped inexplicably in the middle of the road. The man behind the wheel is slumped forward, blue and not breathing, the car still in drive but with his foot on the brake. We revive him with naloxone, and on the way to the hospital, he tells us this is the first time he has used in two months. He is sixty-two years old and says he should know better. He says he is fortunate for deciding to snort a bag while driving rather than pulling over and injecting, which might have killed him. He is apologetic: "I'm sorry for wasting your time. I know you have better things to do." He says he has no excuses for his behavior. When I ask him how he got started, he says he was twelve years old when he got addicted to cough syrup containing codeine. For fifty years he has struggled with opioids.

It is early in the morning when I notice a tall, thin young woman with glasses standing in the rain holding a "homeless and hungry" sign. I recognize her as the girl new to the area whom I had talked with briefly a few days before when my partner Bryan and I were parked in the ambulance across from Pope Park, where we watch users walk east up Park Street and sometimes engage them in conversation. She had come up and asked for cold water, which she heard we carried. She told me her name was Chloe, and she thanked us for the water and a Red Delicious apple I gave her. Now, I have Bryan pull a U-turn so we can talk to her, and I roll down the window as he stops the ambulance at the curb.

"Chloe, right?" I say. "How's it going?"

"Yeah, I'm really sick this morning. I'm not doing too well."

"Sorry we haven't picked up any fruit yet. I have some change." I usually carry some dollar bills in my shirt pocket to give to the homeless, but this time I have to dig into my pants pocket. I pull out a handful of change, maybe $1.70 or so. She thanks us, and we wish her to feel better. That afternoon, she comes by and thanks us again.

I see her again the next day by the shopping plaza. She is trying on a pair of pink high-top sneakers that someone has given her. They are worn and a little too big for her feet, but they make her look oddly stylish. The pink adds color to a black and white day. We exchange small talk, and then I ask her the question: "How did you get started using opioids?"

"My mother was fourteen when I was born," she says. "She gave me up when I was still too little to remember her. I grew up wanting to try heroin. I wanted to know what it was about heroin that would make my mother care more about it than me. I was seventeen when I first tried it. As soon as I used it, I understood."

Parents who use in front of their kids need our mercy. They suffer from the disease of addiction. They can no longer make rational decisions or act with their hearts. Opioids have rewired their reward pathways.

When I was a kid, we saw a movie in science class in which a little man sat in a person's brain and operated a control panel that helped the person choose an apple and know that it tasted good. Years later, the same idea was the premise for the animated movie *Inside Out*, in which various characters representing different emotions vie for command of the brain console that governs a young girl's actions. In the case of a heroin user, picture a home invasion in the brain. The door to the control room is kicked down, and a skeletal figure charges in, roughly pushes the mother away from the brain panel, and seizes control. We may not approve of the actions the new operator now takes, but we can't forget about the mother lying wounded in the corner. She is still in there and needs our help.

Stigma

Stigma is defined as "a mark of shame or discredit: STAIN."[1] It is synonymous with disgrace, dishonor, ignominy, and humiliation. The stigma of being an "addict" implies that you are to blame for your actions. It suggests not just moral judgment against you, but it also inspires fear in others, works to isolate you, and both criminalizes and patronizes your behavior. The user becomes a stereotype and not a person. You are a dope fiend, not someone considered capable of human interaction.

When I tell people I engage with heroin users, many warn me to be careful. They see flashing danger signs. Shouldn't I fear being knifed in an alley or beaten and robbed? When I tell them that I know a homeless heroin user named Luke, who is teaching me how to spin a basketball on my finger, and that one day I brought my ten-year-old daughter to meet him and paid him to give us basketball-spinning lessons, they are aghast. How could I expose her to such a person?

I think for many there is both fear of the unknown and perhaps a belief that the problem of the opioid epidemic is beyond the scale of any one person to make a difference, so what they see before them is a societal problem rather than a person. Instead of seeing someone in need who could be their neighbor, they see danger. Like the parable of the Good Samaritan teaches, how we treat strangers is a test for our heart and character. Will this person rob me? Am I putting myself in danger? Should I pass to the other side of the street? Rather than walk away, I see an opportunity to treat a fellow human as I would wish myself, my family, or my friends to be treated. Rather than look away, I will have compassion for this soul. I will raise water to his lips. I will see that his wounds are bound up. I will be a neighbor unto him.

There is a concept called the three *D*s of stigma: difference, danger, and discrimination. Difference is about keeping drug users out of normal society. Danger is about keeping drug users away from others. Discrimination is about keeping drug users down, denying them opportunities available to the rest of society. The three *D*s isolate and oppress drug users.[2]

In a workbook on drug-related stigma put together by the National Harm Reduction Coalition, I read a quote from Steven Biko, the great South African human rights leader, who said, "The most potent weapon of the oppressor is the mind of the oppressed." If you can destroy a man's self-worth, you can cripple his ability to stand up.[3]

When we in EMS shame patients for using drugs after we revive them, we only further the stigma and drive them farther away from the self-confidence they need to attempt recovery. A man is homeless. He's lost his job and his family. He doubts his worth as a man. And now he is in full-scale drug withdrawal. He is sick and nauseated and wonders if he will ever be well again. Instead of receiving compassion from those sent to help him, he has health care workers berating him for his actions. Why wouldn't he want to go back out again and use a drug that provides him with a temporary sanctuary from the hell his life has become, a drug that enables him to forget for a while his sorrows and pain?

I know first responders who adopt the tough approach with these patients like I used to do: "What's wrong with you? Quit abusing yourself! Get your act together, man. Think of your family. I'm just trying to help you here with what I'm saying. Do you want to remain an addict and end up dead, or do you want to contribute to society and make something of your life?" They think they are helping with the tough-love lecture, but I know now the damage those words can do.

To counter stigma, there has been a considerable effort to educate people about what language to use for the opioid crisis.[4] The word *abuse* is an example of a word that can be damaging. It suggests that the person's condition is the result of willful misbehavior. People with lung disease are not known as cigarette abusers. People with obesity-related disease are not known as food abusers. People injured in car accidents are not known as vehicle abusers. But people who use drugs are branded abusers. *Abuse* calls to mind actions deserving of punishment.

When I encountered my first heroin "addicts," I knew them as substance abusers. I didn't realize it, but I walked onto the scene already prejudging them. I was tired and overworked and there I was because the "addict" who'd caused this 911 call had chosen to abuse drugs. This precipitated a different response in me than would the "victim" of a car crash whose life was suddenly turned upside down by an unanticipated "accident." Car crash victims don't deliberately stick a dirty needle into a vein and push in an "illegal" drug they know could potentially kill them. Even today, when we in EMS fill out our patient care reports, we must choose from a drop-down menu of medical conditions that includes "Substance Abuse" and "Motor Vehicle Accident." I can see clearly now why many of us are programmed to treat drug users differently from other patients who suffer from diseases not stigmatized.

In his essay "The Rhetoric of Recovery Advocacy: An Essay on the Power of Language," William L. White, an addiction and recovery expert, writes, "For more than two centuries, addicted and recovering people in America have been the object of language created by others. People experiencing severe and persistent alcohol and other drug problems have inherited a language not of their own making that has been ill suited to accurately portray their experience to others or to serve as a catalyst for personal change."[5]

In 2015, the Office of National Drug Control Policy releases a list of suggested language to characterize drug use. Here are some of them: Instead of "dirty," say "actively using." Say "regular substance use" instead of "drug habit." Use "person in recovery" instead of "reformed addict."

Earlier in my career I can imagine what I would have said to someone who tried to convince me of the need to change the language I use: "Say 'person who uses drugs' rather than 'junkie,' 'addict,' or 'scumbag.'" To this I'd roll my eyes and answer, "As a writer, I use simple descriptive words to get my points across. A man uses heroin; he is both a junkie and a scumbag." I, of course, would have been lacking both the education in addiction back then—the cumulative experience of listening to my patients' stories and understanding how they came to find themselves where they are—and the vision to see how stigma impairs a person's ability to recover. If this proponent of new language had talked to me and I had answered in such a flippant way, I would like to think he would have slapped the back of my head and said, "You are better than that. This is serious. Pay attention and learn."

The point is that words matter. They can carry judgments, and those judgments affect people, which can create barriers to progress. Stigma can cause people to avoid seeking treatment. The negative view of drug use in society can make users feel even worse about their plight, causing them shame, anxiety, and depression, often propelling them deeper into drug use to dull their feelings. A person using drugs who seeks help at a hospital and is judged negatively in the emergency room will not go back. That person will remember being stigmatized. That was true for a user named Annie.

I talk to Annie, who has a nasty abscess in the crook of her arm that is dirty and infected. "You've got to go to the ED and have that looked at," I say. "I think it's past just putting ointment on it."

"They treat us like shit there. I'll never go back. No one out here will go there unless they absolutely have to."

"Your abscess is getting to that point."

She shakes her head. I try to tell her that there are good and compassionate people at the ED who will help her, but she has been scarred by those who didn't. The last thing she wants is to be judged. She has had enough lectures, and the lectures don't work. She needs kindness and no judgment. Instead, her past treatment has thrown up roadblocks to the care she desperately needs.

But getting rid of stigma is not easy. And too often first responders feed stigma rather than decrease it.

"Listen," an officer says, pointing his finger in the face of a man who has just been revived with naloxone. "You are either a criminal doing a criminal activity, in which case you are going to jail, or you are a victim of a disease, in which case you are going to the hospital. You choose. Criminal or victim? Squad car or ambulance?"

I just shake my head. While many of Hartford's police officers show remarkable compassion, there are still those, as there are in EMS and in hospitals, who don't yet get it, and it goes back to the lack of education. If we can educate, we can eliminate stigma. If we can eliminate stigma, we can end users' isolation. We can bring them back into our community and help them recover.

We get called for a woman in withdrawal seeking detox. She is at a bus stop with all her belongings stuffed into two large garbage bags. We get her on a stretcher and carry her bags with us to the ambulance. She is aching and has abdominal pain and nausea. It has been twelve hours since she last used. And however bad she is feeling now, she knows it's only going to get worse. "Will they treat me okay there?" she asks me.

"I hope so," I say.

"A couple of the nurses don't like me."

"Maybe they won't be working, and at any rate, even if they are not as nice as they could be, you'll have a place to rest for a little while and can get something to eat."

"I'm not hungry," she says. She looks miserable.

"Well, you can at least rest."

We talk on the way there. I learn that she broke her back in a car accident twenty years ago when she was seventeen. Once her doctor cut her off from Percocet, she bought pills on the street. It took her only nine months to turn to heroin, which has been her captor ever since. She has been on the streets for most of the last fifteen years. She can't remember the number of times she's been in rehab.

When we get to the ED, I go to the triage desk and give my report. The nurse looks over at the woman on our stretcher. "Ah, our friend Carol," she says. "Has she been difficult for you?"

"No, perfectly fine."

The nurse nods. "She was here last week for abdominal pain, looking for pain meds. When I said she had to sit in the waiting room and wait her turn, she went spider monkey on me. Security had to throw her out."

"She's in no shape to fight anyone right now," I say, understanding that sometimes users who are in withdrawal and seeking drugs can let their irritability turn into bad behavior. It is not uncommon to hear users and nurses cuss each other out. The nurses are struggling to place patients without enough beds available, and the users, in the throes of withdrawal, want to stop feeling sick. They want someone to acknowledge the hell going on inside their body. When they get what they perceive as a callous or uncaring response, they can react badly.

I walk with the nurse over to our stretcher. "Remember me," the nurse says to Carol. Two muscled security guards stand behind the nurse with their arms crossed. There is something about the nurse's tone and stance that remind me of a prison warden.

"Oh, fuck," Carol says. "She's the one I was talking about."

"Hello, Carol," the nurse says. "Are you going to behave, or are we going to have to restrain you?"

"I'm sick," Carol says, quietly.

"You know we are awfully busy here today."

"I'm sick," she says again, but more tensely.

I start shaking my head. I have seen this scene play out many times before, and it seems so unnecessary.

"Are you going to sit quietly until it's your turn?"

"Fuck you," Carol says.

The scene quickly deteriorates and ends with Carol tied, screaming, to a bed in four-point restraints.

Sometimes I just stand there and watch it. Sometimes I speak up. One time I am waiting at the hospital with a man on my stretcher who is in full-scale withdrawal. He received too much Narcan from first responders. "I got to use the bathroom," he says. "I'm going to shit myself." He looks at me. I can see his desperation. "Please!"

The hospital doesn't like for us to take our patients off our stretchers until they have been triaged. My preceptee partner is giving our report to the nurse. There is a bathroom just down the hall. "Okay," I say. "Here's the deal. I let you off. Your girlfriend has to go in the bathroom with you, and I stand by the door so it doesn't get locked." He readily agrees, and I wheel the stretcher to the restroom door. I let him down, and he rushes in. A few minutes later, the triage nurse and a husky security guard come toward me, looking quite angry. "He can't be in there. He's got to stay on the stretcher," the nurse says. "He could overdose again."

"His girlfriend is in there with him, and I am keeping the door ajar," I say. "He was going to shit himself."

"You do heroin, you have to deal with the result. That's Narcan for you."

"That's cruelty," I say. "Let him finish." I stand my ground, and they back away. Our patient comes out and gets back on the stretcher. The nurse and the guard escort us to the hospital pod, where we put him in their bed. Nothing more is said.

Withdrawal and Relapse

Many people would think that someone who nearly died of a heroin overdose and had to be revived with naloxone would get scared straight and quit heroin for good. I have heard many heroin users express the exact same sentiment to me after I resuscitated them—the ones, at least, who could admit they used drugs: "I'm never doing this again." "My drug-using days are over." "Fuck! I could have died." "Thank you for saving me."

A police officer suggests to me that if only we could videotape people when they are overdosed and show it back to them so they could see what they looked like—blue and not breathing—then it would scare them straight, and they would never use again. From what I have seen of heroin, I don't think it would matter. Unfortunately, most individuals who swear they will never use again go right back to using.

A sixty-year-old one-legged diabetic man overdoses in his bathroom; a syringe still half-filled with a brown liquid heroin mix lies on the floor next to his walker. After I revive him, he looks me in the eye and says, with all his forty-plus years of drug-using experience, "I ain't doing this shit anymore." Both of his arms are deeply track marked from fingers to elbows. There are even scars on his neck. "You need to have Narcan in your house," I say, not buying his declaration. "I'll show your wife how it works."

Patients who have had a nonfatal overdose are at the highest risk of having a subsequent fatal overdose. A recent study from Brigham and Women's Hospital in Massachusetts showed that one out of ten people who were given naloxone outside the hospital by EMS responders (and who survived for at least one day) died within a year, according to statewide medical records.[1] Naloxone will save a person's life in the moment, but unless there is further and effective intervention, this population remains at extreme risk.

When patients are brought to the hospital after an overdose, they are generally watched for a couple of hours and then discharged home, as long as they are alert and oriented. Heroin users tell me that a heroin high typically lasts six to eight hours. Although its full potency declines quickly, heroin remains in the user's system for hours. By the sixth hour they may start to feel withdrawal symptoms if they are regular users. Naloxone does not last as long as heroin or other opioids do. The half-life of naloxone is only sixty to ninety minutes, and it is often redistributed away from the brain, diminishing its functional use.[2] There is a fear that someone revived with naloxone could later return to an overdosed state and die if left alone. In reality, this rarely happens, unless someone has taken a long-acting opioid pill. If they stay alert after the naloxone has worn off, and their oxygen saturation is normal, they are considered safe to discharge.[3]

Discharged overdose patients are often sent out the ED doors with a xeroxed sheet of paper listing area treatment programs, many of which have long waiting lists. Compare this to a patient who's admitted for observation after suffering a mild heart attack or a mini-stroke; this patient is immediately enrolled in a cardiac or stroke rehab program that has no waiting list. True, many opioid overdose patients aren't interested in getting treatment, particularly since the craving that brought them to overdose in the first place remains unabated. But for those who do want help, a speedy path to a facility that can help them is often not available, and they are forced to fend for themselves.

A research letter published in the *Journal of the American Medical Association* in October 2015 found that 78 percent of opioid-dependent people in American were not in treatment.[4] An article in the *American Journal of Public Health* two months earlier found a nationwide shortage of almost a million treatment slots if everyone addicted sought help.[5]

Most opioid users whom medics revive with naloxone and bring to the hospital are sent home or back to the street within hours of their arrival, if they don't leave against medical advice before they are even discharged. In Hartford, 88 percent of opioid overdose patients who are transported to the hospital are discharged home from the emergency department, most in less than two or three hours after their arrival.[6] Patients who are alert and oriented have the right to leave. Those who stay long enough to get discharge instructions may get one simple instruction: stop using heroin.

I am not kidding. That is the extent of the instructions, in all caps: STOP USING HEROIN.

Many overdose patients, once revived, are subjected to less-than-compassionate treatment from both emergency responders and hospital staff. They may already have shame and contempt for themselves and the behavior they can't control. Is it any wonder that these same people—who have just used heroin because they were dope sick or were driven to it by compulsion and who then have that high replaced with withdrawal by Narcan—will go right back out and use again despite the emphatic discharge instruction?

Opioid withdrawal is commonly described as having the worst flu ever, the flu times one thousand. Withdrawal is the opposite of getting high. Instead of bliss and euphoria, the patient can expect anxiety, sweats, nausea, vomiting, abdominal cramping, diarrhea, and tremendous body aches. Some say they do heroin only to keep from being sick. They have long abandoned the quest to relive that first great high.

Most opioid users will do anything to avoid withdrawal, which they face every day unless they get their next dose. That means getting a fix every six to eight hours for heroin users and every three to four hours for those who are using fentanyl, which doesn't last as long as heroin. Even the thought of not being able to obtain their next fix can cause extreme anxiety.

"I just want a few stitches and then I am out of there," says a man who is splattered with blood from head to toe. He holds his arm up in the air, the tourniquet applied tightly above his elbow, a trauma dressing wrapped around his forearm where the first responder told me there was arterial bleeding. The man said he put his arm through glass while working on cleaning up a work site. "How long is this going to take?" he asks with great agitation. "I don't have all day. I've got to get back to work. The cops are not going to be involved, are they?"

"No, they shouldn't be," I say.

"Good, because I work under the table. How come the lights and sirens aren't on? Why are we sitting here?"

"The hospital is just a couple blocks away. I'm calling them now so they will be ready."

"Hurry up already. Christ! I just want them to stitch me up so I can get out of there. Last time I fractured my skull, I was there all fucking day."

"They'll have to examine you first, and then that will decide how long you'll be there."

"If it takes too long, I'm leaving."

I am sensing that his agitation comes from a fear of going into drug withdrawal. He fits the profile. Disheveled thirty-five-year-old male, skinny, tattoos, working off the books at a questionable job site just blocks from Park Street, where the city's drug trade is thriving. He's not in withdrawal now, but he was close to getting enough cash to buy a few bags before the sickness hit. Now, not only does he have no money on him; he is also not going to be in a position to score. As much as he hopes his wound might be nothing, he knows he is covered in blood. If he hadn't applied pressure over the spurting blood and lifted his arm up in the air, he could have bled to death before the first responders could even fit the tourniquet on him.

Still, he can't wait for the sickness to grab him. He's got to get back to the job site, get his money, and get his bags: "Fuck! How come we're not moving any faster!"

In the hospital trauma room, he is surrounded by gowned staff. I can see in his eyes the growing panic. "I just need a few stitches," he says. "I need to get back to work. Now!"

When they release the tourniquet, the blood spurts to the ceiling before they can tighten it again. He isn't going anywhere soon.

I see Chloe on the street, and as with other users, I try to gauge her readiness for recovery. I sense she's ready. In addition to using heroin, she has been supporting herself through sex work—no easy living.

"I'm ready. I'm tired of this life," she says.

"Hop in back," I say. "We'll take you over to Saint Fran, and they'll get you into treatment. Today's the day."

"I'm going to do it. Can you pick me up in an hour?"

"How about right now? We're right here. The door's open."

She fidgets. "I'm sick," she says. "I'm going to go do just one bag. I just, I just can't. I'm worried I'm going to be sick at the hospital. Let me do one bag and then meet me here in an hour."

"How about we take you over there now? Saint Francis has a Suboxone program. As soon as you go into withdrawal, they'll give you some Suboxone, and that'll ease your distress. They'll get you in a program. How about it?"

"I just need to do one bag. Come back for me in an hour. I need to be feeling good when I go there. I can't wait there and be sick."

"Okay," I say. But an hour later, she is nowhere to be found.

The same scene plays out between me and other users many times. Users want to get help because many truly do want a new start, but the fear of being sick in the hospital and having no one to pay them any attention is too great to overcome. It's a river that is hard for them to cross. I imagine a day when I can get Chloe in the back of the ambulance and call into medical control for an order to give her a dose of Suboxone myself—or even, imagine this, medical heroin like they have in England. The drug would tide her over and get her across that bridge to a chance at a new life.

We're sent to the courthouse, where a marshal takes us back to a holding cell. A thin bearded man with cuffs around his wrists and chains on his legs is bent over in the bare cell, grimacing. "Guess he got nervous about seeing the judge," the marshal says to us, "and developed himself some back pain."

"I've had back pain all day," the man says. "And I'm not ducking anything. I'm in here for panhandling, for chrissake. I can't fucking sit up."

"You didn't tell that to the officer who brought you here?"

"He knew I had pain. I was sitting on the side of the road, holding my sign. I couldn't even stand up. He had to help me into the goddamned squad car. He brought me right here. I've got a warrant for failure to appear for another panhandling charge. Big bad criminal, that's me."

There is a term, *jailitis*, which refers to prisoners faking sickness to get out of jail. They know they have to be taken to the hospital for an evaluation if they have a serious medical complaint, and even though they know they'll be taken back to their cell eventually, the trip to the hospital breaks up the monotony of their time in confinement. It is so common that jailors tend to disbelieve that anyone locked in a cell and complaining of poor health could ever be sincere about their condition. The jail calls us, per policy, only to avoid liability, should anyone be truly sick and not get care.

"I'm in terrible pain right now," the man says to the marshal. "I'm always in pain but not this bad. Plus, in another hour, I'm going to be puking and shitting myself."

We transport the man with one hand cuffed to the stretcher railing and a police officer following us in a squad car. The prisoner tells me his tale. He is from a town down on the shore and comes up to Hartford to buy fentanyl. He says he hurt his back in a construction accident ten years ago. He went to a pain doctor, who over time increased his pain prescription to three 80 mg oxycodones a day. "Then one day I go in, and his receptionist tells me he got arrested," the man says. "No other doctor would take me. I'm on three 80 mg oxycodones, for chrissake! What choice did I have then? Just stop taking it?" He shakes his head. "Let me tell you. You don't ever want to go through withdrawal. I'll do anything to avoid it."

He is only forty-two but looks like he's in his late fifties. His face is hard and deeply lined. His tortured blue eyes look like he knows what it is to be chained in a dungeon. He reminds me of the character in *The Far Side* cartoons who is always chained to a wall. The difference is that this man is real, and nothing about his condition is funny. "Withdrawal—it's fucking hell," he says.

Detoxing from heroin can take three days to a week. A patient who goes it alone, known as quitting "cold turkey," is in for a very unpleasant time. People who go to detox centers can get pharmaceutical-aided withdrawal, which, depending on the method, can take from four hours to four weeks, as they are given milder opioids such as methadone and Suboxone to ease their cravings. Once people have gone through withdrawal and are finally starting to feel well again, they may never return to the way they were before using the drug, despite the fact that heroin is gone from their system. Detoxed drug users are not cured of addiction. For many, particularly longtime users, the damaged wiring in their brain remains.

Off heroin for a year, most former users still think about using. The rewired reward center in their brain is still firing its signals: *I need to get heroin. I need to get heroin.* Just the thought of heroin reminds them of those fireworks they used to feel when they used. Every day, every week, every month, every year, the ex-user continues to thinks about it. Triggers from the past increase the desire:[7] driving down Park Street and passing the bakery where he used to meet his dealer to buy heroin; hearing U2's "It's a Beautiful Day," the song she was listening to when she first snorted heroin; seeing Bobby, an old friend he used with; or walking out of the dollar store and seeing an empty heroin bag on the ground stamped "Stardust."

When a former user encounters a trigger, the brain lights up with chemical signals that summon up the past. *You know you want it. You know how good it feels. Things aren't going well for you right now. Nobody loves you like I love you. Wouldn't it be nice to feel that way again? Just try me, just one time.* Fireworks go off at the memory of it. *Let's get together. We'll just talk. No one will know. It would be good to see you again.* The drugs are always there, waiting. Every single day. The lure follows ex-users through every door and is there waiting on the other side. Life not going well? Need an escape? Heroin is the ever faithful friend who loves till death do you part.

Once the brain is rewired, the result may be permanent for many. Even those who have not used for more than a decade can never let their guard down; their relationship with opioids will always be precarious. Addiction is a chronic disease, always capable of coming back.

My partner and I are driving toward Saint Francis Hospital and Medical Center when we see a young man walking down the street in blue jeans and a hospital gown. It is not a completely unfamiliar sight. While patients sometimes go AWOL from the hospital, many are discharged with nothing on but a hospital gown, particularly if they came to the hospital without a full set of clothes or had their clothes cut off by EMS to expose their chest or limbs in order to insert an IV or place the leads of an electrocardiograph.

A half an hour later our radio goes off: "911. Fifty-three Albany Avenue. Priority one, unresponsive."

"I think that's Subway," I say, as Jerry acknowledges the call on the radio.

We arrive just as the fire department is unlocking the bathroom door. Inside, a young man wearing a hospital gown is prone on the ground, stiff like he's having a seizure, except there is no jerking. His eyes are open, but he is not seeing. Drool comes from his mouth. He is purple. I see a syringe on the ground and several torn heroin envelopes. After turning him over, the fire department EMTs get out an Ambu bag and start bagging him. I hit him with 1.2 milligrams of Narcan in his thigh. The tension in his muscles releases, but he is still not breathing better than a couple times a minute. His level of carbon dioxide is lethally high at 92, which means he is not ventilating, not getting rid of the carbon dioxide building up in his lungs. We place an oral airway in his mouth to make bagging easier by keeping his tongue from occluding his breathing passage. "Look at this," I say, pointing to the Saint Francis Hospital bracelet around his wrist. It shows his name and the date of admission to the ED. It's today.

The young man coughs, spits out the airway, and wakes with a start.

"Easy, easy," I say. "You OD'd."

"I did not. I'm fine."

"Seriously," I say.

"Fuck," he says.

"Back to Saint Fran?"

He tells me his story. He got out of jail this morning and went right to lower Albany Avenue. He bought a syringe at the bodega on Mather for two dollars and then a bag of heroin at Albany and Center for four. He left Saint Francis against medical advice and did the same thing.

"I'm just going to get out and do it again," he says. "They just need to send me back to jail. It's the only place I am safe."

"If you were clean and not in withdrawal, why did you feel such a need to use?" I ask.

"You don't understand," he says. "I'm an addict. I can't help it. I need to be locked up. I'm safe in jail. I told the cop to arrest me. I'm going to die out here."

In most states, opioid users who go to jail have to go through forced detox; what is more, they are offered no help for their addiction. Even patients who are on a methadone or Suboxone regime prescribed by a doctor are denied these essential drugs while they are incarcerated. And they receive no therapy to help them cope with the inevitable triggers to use they will face when they return to their old environment. Is it any wonder they so easily fall back into using?

We find a semi-responsive man, vomiting on his kitchen floor. We are in Bloomfield, a suburb of Hartford, in a new housing development in the north end of the town. I am struck by how nice the house is, with its hardwood floors and expansive windows, but also by how barren it is. The large living room has only a sofa, arm-chair, and TV. The dining room is empty. There is only a small table with two chairs in the kitchen. The man is on the floor next to the table, and he is groggy. He is a muscled man in his forties, with a lined, weather-beaten face. His wife, a professional woman in business dress, came home from work, found him barely re-sponsive, and called 911.

She tells us that he recently had shoulder surgery and is on blood thinners for clots in his legs. She has no idea what has hap-pened or how long he has been there. When we arrive, we find he can barely answer questions. He is not hurt, his grips are equal, he has no facial droop or other sign of stroke, but his speech is slow. He looks at his wife and says he's sorry. I ask what pain meds he is on. I'm thinking he took too many and maybe drank some alcohol, although I smell no liquor on his breath.

We get him up on the stretcher, and as we start out the door, I suddenly hear the wife say, "Hold on a minute." She has found something in the bathroom: heroin. She is so angry that she's be-side herself, she tells us. The officer asks her if this is something he regularly does.

"No. He's been clean for almost sixteen years—since before I met him. He's been up front about his past with me, but I've never seen it. He doesn't even drink. I can't believe he did this. I could kill him."

"It's the most addictive drug in the world," the officer says. "No one ever completely beats it."

"I just can't believe this. I'm in shock."

She comes to the hospital with us, riding in the front. "Is he okay?" she asks.

"He's stable," I say. "He'll be all right."

She cries. "He's been so depressed," she says. "He lost his grown son two weeks ago. He's been out of work with his injury.

He's had no money. We have a new home, and with him not working, we can't afford to put anything in it."

"He's beaten this before," I say. "He can do it again. Don't be too hard on him. It sounds like he's had a rough go."

"I could just kill him," she says, but not as harsh this time.

After we leave them in an ED room, I come back later and glance in. She sits next to his bed, leaning against him, her head against his shoulder, his big arm around her. He brushes her hair. Neither of them speaks.

The sad fact is that while MRI brain scans have shown that some people's brains can recover from addiction, the lure of heroin imprinted in the cells through damaged reward pathways is so strong that relapse is expected for a great many former users. Victory is measured not in complete cure but in time still alive on earth.

A girl is sprawled on a couch, and a firefighter is bagging her. She gets naloxone up the nose, and a few minutes later, with a little sternal rub, she opens her eyes.

"You overdosed," the firefighter says.

She shakes her head and slowly sits up. "I'm so embarrassed," she says.

She is in her early thirties and looks striking, like the actress Scarlett Johansson, except she has hard miles on her face and is a heroin addict. The firefighter says she overdosed yesterday too. They found her in a car on Williams Street.

"I am so sorry," she says. "I was clean for four months, and I relapsed yesterday. And here I am again. I'm sorry."

I notice her boyfriend is also in the room. He is a tall burly man with a beard. He is clearly high on heroin himself. His pupils are pinpoint, and he speaks in an odd whispery voice. He is unsteady in the knees. He says they are from out of town but know the person whose apartment we are in. The boyfriend shot her up in the stairwell before they went to the man's apartment, not wanting to involve him in their addiction. When she stopped breathing, he called 911 on his cell phone. After getting the man to help, they carried her into the man's apartment. The boyfriend says he bought the drugs on Park Street.

The girl still has her head in her hands. "I have to be at work at ten," she says.

A police officer is there and wants to know where the syringe is. The boyfriend says he left it in the stairwell. "Where a kid can find it!" the officer says.

"I'm sorry. I panicked. I needed to get her help," he says.

They go off to find the syringe. The girl stands slowly and walks out of the apartment with us, over to a small elevator, which we take to the ground floor, where my partner has the stretcher set up.

I am thinking she looks familiar to me. I remember now where I saw her. She overdosed in the Subway bathroom last summer on the Fastrack brand. She was on the ground, blue and agonal (labored, gaspy breathing). We brought her around with Narcan. I remember her being very apologetic. We had a conversation about the brands. She wanted to know which ones were most dangerous (the ones with fentanyl) so she could avoid them. "Stay away from Fastrack," I'd told her.

"Lesson learned," she'd said.

On the way to the hospital, I ask her now how she first got involved with opioids. I am expecting her to tell me, as so many do, that she got into a car accident or was injured somehow. Instead she says, "I don't remember. I'm an addict. I've always been an addict. It's who I am."

We ride along in silence. I try to think about what I can say to make her feel better about herself. It seems she's had all her self-worth beaten out of her by the turns her life has taken and likely by having so many people stigmatize her that she came to believe them.

"If I don't get to work by ten, I am going to lose my job," she says. She is a waitress at an all-night diner several towns over off Interstate 84. It's six-thirty now. A couple of hours in the ED, and she may get out in time.

"Don't give up hope," I say.

Heartache

In Homer's *Odyssey*, the Greek hero Odysseus and his men—worn out from the ten-year Trojan War, filled with sadness for the loss of comrades, and beaten down by their long and difficult journey homeward—come to the island of the Lotus Eaters, where the inhabitants offer them a special plant to eat to ease their sorrow. Eating the lotus enables Odysseus's men to forget their heartaches. They lose all desire to continue their journey home.[1] In "The Lotos-eaters," a poem by Alfred Lord Tennyson about the same tale, the Greek men beg the world to "let us alone." They welcome the lotus's power to make them forget. "Give us long rest or death, or dreamful ease," they beg.[2] In one of the first interventions recorded in literature, Odysseus drags them back to the boats and restrains them; then those of his men who avoided the drug row fast, making their escape.

Unfortunately, the lotus of myth has never been limited to a distant island; it is all around us, in every community, and its power has only grown. There have been humans addicted to the opium poppy as long ago as at least 5000 BC. Ancient Sumerians knew opium as the "joy plant." Statues of the Greek gods of sleep, night, death, and love show them adorned with poppies.[3] People use opium and its modern byproducts of morphine and heroin because opioids make them feel better. They bring, if only for a short time, happiness and forgetting of life's sorrow.

But people today weren't given opioids by a strange tribe of Lotus Eaters. In fact, many received them from licensed health care professionals who sincerely believed they were doing right by their patients. Others received them from coworkers, friends, or acquaintances who promised the pills would help cure their ailing.

I don't ask my patients why they use opioids; I ask them how they got started. Many, like the young cheerleader of chapter 4, got hurt or sick. They were in car crashes or suffered athletic injuries or had painful medical conditions or surgeries. Their doctors prescribed them the opioids Percocet or OxyContin, often with prescriptions extending to six months. They were told to take them as needed. While opioids affect each person differently, the pills make some feel like nothing they have ever known. The pills fill a hole they didn't know they had. The pills relieve not just their physical pain but their hidden emotional pain as well. They feel happy. Some get addicted and suffer sickness when their prescription runs out or they can no longer obtain the pills from their friend. They start buying pills on the street. And they soon learn that heroin is much cheaper and more widely available and works even better than the pills. Like Homer's men in the land of the Lotus Eaters, the drugs take over their lives.

The results are horrific, both on a national and personal scale. More Americans are now dying each year from opioids than died in the entire Vietnam War. According to statistics from the American Society of Addiction Medicine, 2.5 million Americans are addicted to prescription opioids or heroin.[4] Jobs and homes are lost; families are destroyed. The economic costs are estimated to exceed $500 billion dollars between 2018 and 2020, according to a report by the Altarum health research group.[5]

Those are powerful figures I would put into a speech if I were still working for a United States senator or state governor. But even such high numbers lack the power of the stories of the epidemic's victims.

Shelly worked in a restaurant. She was a twenty-eight-year-old single mom who was going through a hard time. Her daughter's father had left them. She was staying with her mother and step-dad, who she felt were always judging her negatively. She noticed that one of her coworkers was happy all the time, no matter what was going on in his life. She asked him why that was. He said he used heroin. So Shelly tried it with him one night. And she had never felt so good. All her cares went away.

Three years later, I am taking her from jail to the hospital for nausea. She was arrested for missing a court date on a theft charge. She no longer lives with her mother and stepfather, who have custody of her child. The address she gives me is different from the one on the police booking sheet, different from the one in our computer (she is a repeat patient), and different from the one on the hospital face sheet. She moves about. She says she was on methadone for a while. Methadone is a milder, longer-acting opioid than heroin that is frequently prescribed to users to get them off the stronger, deadlier heroin. Methadone blunts their cravings and lasts up to two days. Users go to a clinic every morning to receive their dose. People on methadone are often able to hold jobs and be functioning members of society. The methadone was working for her, but she didn't have insurance and wasn't on Medicaid yet. They charged her $65 a week, and when she fell behind, they kicked her out of the program. She went back to injecting heroin. She has recently gotten back on Medicaid and hopes to get back on methadone. She says heroin still makes her feel great, though not quite as happy as she had first felt. She regrets trying it. She is tired of living like this. "I used to be a normal person before this all started," she says.

Eric is a twenty-nine-year-old. He broke both his legs in a motorcycle accident four years ago. He was in the hospital for seven weeks. He took pills for the pain, and his doctor kept upping his dose, until one day, two years later, he cut him off completely, telling him he shouldn't be in pain anymore. We find Eric overdosed at a bus stop in downtown Hartford. He wakes and looks up at me in the ambulance. After throwing up, he tells me he has been to rehab three times. He says he's been clean for two weeks, but he slipped up today. "My wife just filed for divorce," he says. "I want to go back to rehab. This is the last time I will use. Enough is enough."

Unfortunately for Eric, as Australian author Luke Davies said about heroin in the novel *Candy*, "When you can stop, you don't want to, and when you want to stop, you can't."[6] We will revive Eric again three weeks later when he is found overdosed in the restroom of the Hartford Public Library.

Tom says he started using pain pills when he was eleven years old. He hung out with an older crowd who drank beer and smoked marijuana and took pills they'd stolen from their parents, who had multiple pain pill prescriptions. He used heroin for the first time at fifteen. He's twenty-three now and living under Interstate 84. While he has tried methadone and Suboxone, the lure of heroin has always been too strong. "I think about it all the time," he says. "That first feeling is so good. It's like nothing you'll ever experience. You just want it. You want it again." He has no plans to stop being an addict: "I know it's going to kill me, but I can't imagine living without it."

Ervin is fifty-eight years old and has been doing heroin since the late seventies. I am taking him to detox from the hospital. He tells me that he got into heroin recreationally with his friends. They partied every weekend—booze, weed, coke—and then one weekend one of his buddies brought along a friend who had heroin. Three of Ervin's friends from that first night had died of heroin overdoses over the years, but Ervin has been careful. Instead of graduating to injecting, which they did, Ervin snorts his heroin and tries not to get too greedy. He is cautious, particularly with the powerful synthetic opioid fentanyl, which is mixed into so many of the bags of heroin.

"When I get money," he says, "I use heroin until my money runs out, and then I check myself into rehab. I come out clean, and then when I get enough money, I start doing heroin again until I am broke, and then I go back to rehab. It is the only choice I have. It's either rehab or robbing or killing someone to get the money to buy more heroin to feed my habit. I am not a violent man and cannot stomach causing harm to anyone but myself. This is the cycle of my life, and I see no end to it. I love heroin. I am happy when I am high, but I wish heroin had never showed up that night. I wonder what my life would have been like had I never let that demon in. I might have had a wife and a family." He looks me hard in the eye: "Don't ever start."

Katie is a thirty-two-year-old cancer survivor. The Percocets her doctor gave her weren't strong enough to blunt the pain as her tolerance to them grew, so during chemo she would supplement the pills with heroin she obtained from a friend. She had a job as a secretary at an insurance company and was engaged to her boyfriend. Unfortunately, the treatments made her infertile. She found out he was cheating on her. "I confronted him about why he would cheat on me after ten years of being together," she tells me. "I thought he was going to say because she had a fat ass, but he said because she can have children. That devastated me. When I use heroin, I forget about the pain he caused me." She says her doctor is going to help her get on methadone. She uses heroin intravenously now and is having a hard time finding a vein; plus, all the chemicals they put in heroin now to cut it can't be good for her. And she is terrified of fentanyl. She thinks fentanyl is why she overdosed today. She caught a hot spot—a clump that didn't mix evenly. She just wants her old life back and for all the pain to go away.

While many start using opioids to cure their physical pain, I come to realize from listening to stories like Katie's that the drugs are as effective, if not more so, at relieving emotional pain by blocking a person's ability to feel. Heroin makes people feel good; it offers relief, although temporary, from pain, stigma, shame, despair, and an uncertain or scary future.

We are sent to a detox center for a diabetic. Diego is a sixty-year-old with a blood sugar level over 600 (80 to 120 is normal), although he has no complaint yet. He has come to the detox center to kick his heroin habit. But first, because his sugar is so high, he will have to go to the emergency department to get his blood sugar under control before he can be admitted to detox.

"I did three bags of heroin this morning," he tells me, "and then I flushed the rest of the bundle down the toilet and came here."

Diego is a man with deep eyes. He speaks quietly when I ask him how he first got started using. "I spent eighteen years in prison," he says. "When I came out, I saw there was so much suffering in the world. People on the outside are used to it, and they don't see it, but I saw it. That's how I got started. It allowed me to escape and forget about what I was seeing. I've been on and off of it for most of my life. I lost two brothers to heroin and a sister and two cousins to crack cocaine. My father died at ninety last week. He was all I had left. I was lost without him. It was a setback for me. I started using again. But I looked at myself this morning and knew I wouldn't see seventy if I didn't get a hold of myself. I knew it was time for me to come in."

I attend a conference where the featured speaker is Austin Eubanks, a survivor of the Columbine high school shooting.[7] He and his childhood best friend were golfing and fishing buddies. He shows us pictures of the two of them smiling, no idea what fate had in store for them.

In the school library, they hear an odd sound from out in the hallway. Another student says it sounds like gunshots. But they are in a school. Guns aren't allowed in schools. Then more commotion, and a teacher bursts into the library and says, "Everyone get under the tables!" Even with that, they stand around for a moment, thinking, *really?* Then the gunmen, armed with shotguns and automatic weapons, enter the library. His best friend and he hide under a table as the shooters walk through the room systematically executing their fellow students. They are under the last table. His friend is killed instantly, while he is shot in the hand and knee.

He survives only by playing dead. He tells us how he detached himself from the scene. Later, when he is rescued and meets his father, he bursts into tears, the emotion finally ripping through him. But then he is medicated for his injuries. Doctors prescribe him heavy doses of powerful drugs. He is seventeen years old and has never had a beer or smoked marijuana. While his physical pain subsides in a matter of days, his emotional pain is still off the charts. He keeps taking the medicine because it mutes the horror he endured. The pills block the intense memories of what he has been through and the horrible thought of all his slaughtered friends. The pills provide an escape that quickly leads to addiction.

Within a matter of months, he is not only drinking alcohol but, as his tolerance for opioids has increased, is also now using illicit drugs. He uses all these substances for years to manage his emotional pain, which is not addressed by any of his doctors. Because he is able to put a tie on and go to work, he fools people, he tells us, even while his life is unraveling. He uses heroin, methamphetamine, and other drugs to keep his emotional pain at bay and to keep from feeling the sickness of withdrawal. After more than a decade of struggle, he finally finds his path out. He makes it through multiple recoveries and reunites with his son and becomes good friends with his ex-wife. He remarries and has another son. He tells us about the difference between feeling better and being better. He becomes a committed advocate and travels the country, speaking about the opioid epidemic and offering messages of recovery and hope.

Austin Eubanks receives a prolonged standing ovation from the packed conference crowd of nearly three hundred, all people dedicated to battling the epidemic. Three weeks later, I open up the newspaper to see the headline "Columbine Shooting Survivor Found Dead." And there is his name: Austin Eubanks. His family issues a statement: "[Austin] lost the battle with the very disease he fought so hard to help others face."[8]

His death stuns all of us who had heard him speak at the conference. Here was someone who went through hell and came out the other side to educate and inspire. How deep his pain must have been, I think, and how strong the lure of opioids. I wonder if he was using when he spoke to us.[9] Were we fooled because he had a tie on and spoke without slurring his words? But most of all I think about what his life might have been if he had not gone to school on April 20, 1999. Thirty-seven-year-olds die of opioid overdoses daily in this country. How do people think of them? Are they scumbags, abusers, and unclean? Or are they members of our community, people to be cared for and shown love and mercy? How close we all are to having our lives fall apart. The possibilities are there for heroin to knock on any of our doors. For Austin

Eubanks, as for many others, heroin was a solitary island in a sea of pain, physical and emotional. He had washed up on the beach in the land of the Lotus Eaters, where he found welcomed relief but little chance of escaping, little chance for a castaway to journey back home.

If you ask me to name one thing we can do to end the suffering, it is to end the stigma. We were taught growing up that drug users were bad people. We were taught to just say no. Most of us believed that those who did heroin had character flaws. That has been ingrained in many of us. But we have also been taught, either in church or by the example of our families or by basic human decency, to love thy neighbor as thyself. Addiction is a brain disease that could affect anyone. Our lack of education about addiction has allowed us to stigmatize patients, and that stigma has blunted our fundamental decency toward our fellow humans; it has struck fear in us and blinded us to the truth that users are just regular people like any of us. I watched a TV special about heroin use in which the mother of a child suffering from addiction says that neighbors always bring casseroles to families with a member fighting an illness but that no one ever brings a casserole to the family with a member fighting addiction. Families lie to friends about the disease that is ruining the life of someone they love. If we could treat everyone afflicted with addiction without stigma, then we would never banish them from our communities. They would get proper care, medical and social. And they would not die, by the hundreds of thousands, alone and forsaken.

Pain Control

In 1998, Purdue Pharma releases an advertisement to market its drug OxyContin. Doctor Alan Spanos sits behind a desk in what looks like a real medical office and speaks in a reasoned tone: "There's no question that our best, strongest pain medicines are the opioids, but these are the same drugs that have a reputation for causing addiction and other terrible things. Now, in fact, the rate of addiction among pain patients who are treated by doctors is much less than 1 percent. They don't wear out; they go on working. They don't have serious medical side effects. So these drugs, which, I repeat, are our best, strongest pain medications, should be used much more than they are for patients in pain."[1]

His words are false. His lie is lethal.

Opioids have always been among the most addictive substances known to man, but that hasn't stopped people from saying otherwise. When morphine was distilled from opium, it was at first marketed as a cure for opium addiction, and cure opium addiction it did. People switched their addiction to morphine. When heroin was created, it was marketed as a cure for morphine addiction. Its proponents claimed they had removed the addictive molecule. They soon had to admit they were wrong.[2] History repeats itself yet again when Purdue Pharma, which claimed oxy-codone is not addictive, is also eventually forced to admit that its pills are addictive and that it had misled the public. In 2007, the company admits this in court to the tune of a $600 million fine.[3] Unfortunately, the destruction the company unleashed amounts to multiple billions, as do its profits. OxyContin earned Purdue Pharma a revenue of $2.8 billion in the seven years from 1995 and 2001 alone. For good reason, controlled substances are closely monitored by the federal Drug Enforcement Administration (DEA). Yet, unfortunately, in this case the profit motive managed to get the better of public health interests.

When I start as a paramedic in Hartford in 1995, I rarely give pain medicine to my patients. We carry morphine, but in order to ad-minister it to a patient, we have to radio the hospital, talk to an emergency doctor, and get a direct order. My paramedic precep-tor tells me, "I have to hurt by looking at you for me even to think about calling for orders to give you pain medicine." Even then, the order is likely for an amount too small to make much difference. As for the types of pain, narcotics are largely given only for pain in the chest or extremities. Giving morphine for abdominal pain is forbidden for fear that it will mask a patient's symptoms and make diagnosis difficult.

This thinking shifts when the medical establishment under-goes a sea change. Pharmaceutical companies, like Purdue, send out armies of salespeople. The companies hire doctors and donate millions to pain societies they help create. They even give money to the Joint Commission that accredits hospitals. All of this is done to change the way that Americans treat pain.

In EMT school, we learn to take a patient's vital signs. The main vital signs are heart rate (pulse), blood pressure, and respiratory rate. We don't measure the fourth traditional vital sign, tempera-ture, because we don't carry thermometers. Instead, we feel the patient's skin and make a rough determination of cold, cool, normal, or hot. Checking the four vital signs is among the first things we do in our primary assessment of patients. Everyone gets their vitals checked—from a young man with a shotgun wound in the chest to an older woman with a stubbed toe.

One day at Hartford Hospital a sign appears in the triage area, the place where we interact with hospital staff to get a room assignment or simply to transfer a patient from our stretcher to a waiting room. The sign says, "Pain—the 5th vital sign." We are asked to report on a patient's level of pain. Zero represents no pain, and ten represents the greatest pain the patient has ever felt. In time, the pain score becomes mandatory on our run forms. Everyone gets a pain score. The measurement must be taken at least twice during our time with a patient. Not only does each patient get a pain score, but we are also taught that pain is different for each person. If a person rates her pain as ten out of ten, we are to accept that. Facial expressions and vital signs do not correlate with a person's pain. One patient can be as stoic as a soldier, another whining like a child. If they both say their pain is a ten, we accept that and treat it accordingly.

I am driving the ambulance one day, and Dexter Johnson, a paramedic I am training, asks a patient with a sore shoulder what his pain level is. "Ten," the man says, despite no outward sign of distress or injury.

"You don't understand," Dexter says to him. "Ten is like alligator-biting-your-leg-off pain. What is your pain?"

"Ten," the man says.

I nearly drive off the road. According to our guidelines Dexter has little choice but to give the man some medical-grade fentanyl. He succeeds in lowering the man's pain to a nine.

I am complaining about this now, but the fact is, at that time, I am one of those medical educators going around preaching the pain-control message. I even propose the guideline that anyone with pain of four or higher should receive analgesia. But people say to me, "What if the patient is drug seeking?" My response is that I would rather treat ten drug seekers than miss one person with legitimate pain for fear of medicating a drug seeker. I go even further. Besides, I ask, why do drug seekers want pain medicine? BECAUSE THEY ARE IN PAIN! The truth is, of course, a bit more complicated than that. Drug seekers often seek out of a fear that they will run out of pain medicine and so become dreadfully sick.

"I'm allergic to ibuprofen," a man tells me as he lies on my stretcher holding his stomach. He says he has ten out of ten pain. He says he lives in New Britain, a city ten miles to the west, but I pick him up at the state library in Hartford. He looks like he hasn't shaved or bathed for days. He is very polite. He wants to go to one hospital. I suggest the other just to test him, but he says he has had bad experiences there.

I believe he is a drug seeker, but I can't say this with 100 percent certainty. If he is in legitimate pain, I don't want to deny him, so I put in an IV and give him 100 micrograms of fentanyl and 4 milligrams of Zofran for his nausea. He looks much more relaxed; he closes his eyes. When I ask him his pain number, he says it is a nine. "Thank you for treating me decently," he says. I am supposed to give him more medicine, according to protocol, as long as his pain is above four and his blood pressure remains above 100, which it does. But he falls asleep before we get to the hospital, so I hold off.

At the hospital, the nurse tells me he was there three days ago for the same complaint, and they gave him Dilaudid, a potent opioid. The staff later noted in the patient's record that he is on the state's list of people who have shown up at multiple hospitals seeking pain meds.

Oh, well, I think. It is not my job to know the difference and be absolutely right in my decisions. I took away his immediate pain;

now the hospital can deal with his long-term issues and try to get him some help, instead of turning him back out on the street to seek more. I climb on the pain bandwagon with gusto and become one of its highest ministers because the literature I read suggests that pain is woefully undertreated.

In 2011, the Institute of Medicine issues the landmark report *Relieving Pain in America: A Blueprint for Transforming Prevention, Care, Education, and Research.* The report's opening paragraph proclaims, "Protection from and relief of pain and suffering are a fundamental feature of the human contract we make as parents, partners, children, family, friends, and community members, as well as a cardinal underpinning of the art and science of healing." The authors warn that pain "can blunt the human values of joy, happiness, and even human connectedness."[4]

I read as much as I can about pain management and share my new knowledge with any group that will have me speak. Every year at our medical advisory committee meeting, I push for more liberal protocols in our regional EMS guidelines, to the point where today we can give up to 20 milligrams of morphine on standing orders (without having to call a doctor on the radio) or up to 300 micrograms of fentanyl. I fight for us to carry fentanyl, which works much quicker than morphine and provides relief in one to two minutes versus five to ten. I introduce a patient-controlled pain protocol: As long as the patient's pain score is a four or higher, the medic asks the patient, "Would you like more pain medicine?" If the patient says yes, the medic administers it. When I go on calls in the city, I have satisfied patients, and I feel great about myself. I am taking care of people who appreciate it.

In my talks, I quote the great physician and philosopher Albert Schweitzer: "We must all die. But that I can save him from days of torture, that is what I feel as my great and ever new privilege. Pain is a more terrible lord of mankind than even death itself." Not surprisingly, the quote is featured on the website of the American Pain Association.[5]

When speaking, I tell my audiences about the term *oligoanalgesia*, which means an underuse of analgesia. I cite papers finding that only 30 to 63 percent of patients in pain at the ED received analgesia. I cite a study of hip fracture patients in which only 18 percent received analgesia from EMS, while 91 percent received treatment in the ED. I emphasize that those treated in the hospital receive pain management in a mean time of 145 minutes after arrival, while those lucky enough to get it from EMS receive it within 28 minutes of EMS's arrival at the scene.[6]

Most people are familiar with the need for speedy treatment in stroke, heart attack, and trauma. It is why ambulances have lights and sirens. The "golden hour of trauma," early defibrillation, and the phrases "time is muscle" for coronary care and "time is brain" for stroke care are known to all in EMS. I add pain management to the list.

The only purpose of pain, I tell my audiences, is to alert us to our injury and stop us from doing anything that will aggravate it. Your leg is broken; don't walk on it. Your back hurts when you pick up a box; put the box down. You touch a hot burner; take your hand off it. Beyond that, pain becomes destructive. It causes inflammation, hinders healing, and sets off a cascade of physiological changes in the body.

I tell my audiences about pain the complainer: If you happen to drop an anvil on your big toe, your toe is going to call up your brain and say, "Hey, brain. Did you see that? You just dropped an anvil on me. It freaking hurts!" In most cases, the toe will stop hurting eventually, the injury will heal, and everything will go back to the way it was. But that isn't always how it works. Pain, I tell them, isn't just an annoying complainer; it is, in the simple and eloquent words of a 2008 article from the *Journal of Emergency*

Medicine, "physiologically bad."[7] Pain is physiologically bad because it is destructive to the body. Untreated, it damages the immune system, hinders wound healing, rewires the neurological system, and can lead to chronic pain.

Consider this statement from a 2006 emergency medicine textbook, *Pain Management and Sedation*: "Prompt treatment of acute pain may prevent both short- and long-term deleterious consequences and resultant chronic pain syndromes."[8] The concept of pain as physiologically bad and my role in relieving it as a paramedic become clearest to me when I read an article on pre-hospital analgesia and sedation written by R. MacKenzie that appears in the February 2000 issue of the *Journal of the Royal Army Medical Corps*: "The effective management of pain in the pre-hospital environment may be the most important contribution to the survival and long-term well-being of a casualty that we can make. The pre-hospital practitioner has the first and perhaps only opportunity to break the pain cascade."[9]

If I arrive on the scene of a patient with an open ankle fracture who is grimacing in pain, I can treat the patient's pain once I load him into the ambulance or I can wait for the hospital to do it because the hospital is only five minutes away. Or I can treat the patient right now where he lies. I am on the clock. The patient's body is undergoing a "cascade" of changes caused by pain.

Here is the sequence if I treat him on the spot: Deliver fentanyl in the nose through an atomizer. Splint the ankle with a pillow. Get him on the stretcher and into the ambulance. Elevate the broken ankle. Ice. Reassess. Pop in an IV. Administer more fentanyl, this time directly into a vein. Take him to the hospital. Perhaps dose fentanyl once again, right there in the ambulance bay when parked outside the ED doors.

If your patient is singing "Oh, Happy Day," you've done your job, O Vanquisher of Pain. You deserve a high five as much as you would for promptly defibrillating a patient in cardiac arrest. Pain management is not just the humane thing for us to do; it is often physiologically the best thing we can do for the patient.

For those who are concerned that patients can become addicted, I cite a "landmark" Boston University study, a study that forms the basis for Purdue Pharma's claim that opioids addict less than 1 percent of patients who are treated with them. In my talks, I show a slide announcing this disarming fact: out of "11,882 patients who received at least one narcotic preparation" at Boston University Medical Center, "there were only four cases of reasonably well documented addiction in patients who had no history of addiction."

Imagine my surprise years later when I learn the truth behind the study. It isn't a study at all but simply a paragraph, a 101-word letter to the *New England Journal of Medicine*. The senior author, Herschel Jick, had a student of his, Jane Porter, look through data he kept on drug side effects to see how many of the hospital's patients developed addiction. The patients monitored were largely cancer patients who had received small amounts of opioids for a brief term while in the hospital. They wrote a short note about their finding and sent it to a leading medical journal.[10] This modest letter to the editor is then cited by *Time* magazine as a "landmark study" showing that concerns about people becoming addicted to prescription opioids are "unwarranted."[11]

Canadian researchers later publish their own letter in the *New England Journal of Medicine* detailing how that one-paragraph letter has been cited 608 times in medical journals since its publication, with increasing citations after the 1996 introduction of OxyContin. They conclude that the 1980 letter was "heavily and uncritically cited as evidence that addiction was rare with long-term opioid therapy."[12]

"Heavily and uncritically cited . . ." Ouch. I am one of the many who got scammed. I don't like being burned.

I learn another new term, *hyperalgesia*. This refers to patients having a heightened perception of pain from chronic opioid use.

Take a hypothetical example: I pinch you hard and cause you a five out of ten pain, and then after months of opioid use for chronic pain, I pinch you again with the same intensity, but your pain is now a seven. That is hyperalgesia. And apparently hyperalgesia is not a new concept. In 1870, the physician Clifford Allbutt, writing in the medical journal *Practitioner*, observed, "At such times I have certainly felt it a great responsibility to say that pain, which I know is an evil, is less injurious than morphia, which may be an evil." He asked, "Does morphia tend to encourage the very pain it pretends to relieve?" And he concluded, "in the cases in question, I have much reason to suspect that a reliance upon hypodermic morphia only ended in that curious state of perpetuated pain."[13] What happens in hyperalgesia is that the dopamine produced by an opioid in its initial phases of use is so great that over time it begins to inhibit the brain's natural ability to produce its own dopamine.

I begin to question whether medicating patients in chronic pain might not be good for them. While today I still medicate patients with acute pain, I wonder whether I will read someday that the pain cascade theory I have cited is just another theory concocted by the pain lobby.

As I am promoting, advancing, and producing fellow pain management disciples, similarly minded people in other medical professions are doing the same, many of whom are lobbied by the National Pain Foundation and other groups that are heavily funded by the drug companies.[14] Free educational seminars on pain management are held in vacation destinations. Doctors who liberally prescribe pain pills, under the theory that no one should have to live in pain, become patient favorites, and their business picks up. Patients are grateful to doctors who listen and give them prescriptions to ease their suffering. The Joint Commission requires that hospitals survey their patients about their satisfaction with pain management. Hospitals that rate poorly in pain management satisfaction for patients receive less money in federal reimbursement.

Imagine the quandary this puts physicians in. If they fail to relieve their patient's pain, they are subject to a poor evaluation. Administrators in the hospital likely track each physician's pain management score out of concern for the hospital's financial return.[15] Doctors who cost the hospital money by failing to medicate patients' pain fully could find themselves out of a job. (Fortunately, this practice later changes. While surveying for patient pain satisfaction still occurs, it no longer carries a financial penalty.)[16] In July 2019, Congress asks the American Pain Society and nine other organizations, including the Joint Commission, to disclose their financial relationships with opioid manufacturers.[17] The American Pain Society soon shutters its doors in light of the multiple lawsuits it is facing for its role in the epidemic.[18]

According to the National Survey on Drug Use and Health, conducted between 2011 and 2013, studies show that people hooked on prescription pills are forty times more likely to get addicted to heroin.[19] You get injured, you go to a doctor, and she gives you a six-month prescription for Percocet to take as needed for pain. Some people don't like the way the pills make them feel, so they stop taking them as soon as the acute pain goes away. They flush them down the toilet or stow the bottle in the medicine cupboard along with other old prescriptions to be forgotten about unless needed. But other people are more genetically disposed to the pills, and they take them as prescribed or maybe even a few more than indicated per day because they drive the pain away and make them feel so good.

The problem with opioids is that the body adapts to them quickly and builds up a tolerance. A person takes the same number of pills, but the effect is less. That person needs more pills to feel the same way. No problem. The doctor writes another prescription for a stronger version. The cycle continues until the person's need outruns the prescription or until the doctor cuts back on the amount or cuts the patient off completely.

While Purdue Pharma claimed that less than 1 percent of patients who are prescribed opioids become addicted, a 2015 research study and literature review in the journal *Pain* finds that 21 to 29 percent of patients prescribed opioids for chronic pain misuse them and 8 to 12 percent become addicted.[20]

Just how many people in America are prescribed pain pills? More people in this country are prescribed pain pills than use tobacco products. In 2012, according to the National Prescription Audit, Connecticut has 72 pain prescriptions for every 100 people. In Alabama, there are 143 pain prescriptions for every 100 people.[21] By 2017, in Connecticut, the number of opioid prescriptions is down to 48 per 100 people, a decline of 30 percent. The national rate in 2017 is 58.7. Over that same period, however, the opioid death rate rises from 1.6 deaths per 100,000 persons in Connecticut to 7.7 deaths, an almost five-fold increase.[22]

Opioid users can become addicted quickly. A 2017 study in the *Morbidity and Mortality Weekly Report*, prepared by the Centers for Disease Control and Prevention, finds that "the probability of long-term opioid use increases most sharply in the first days of therapy, particularly after 5 days or 1 month of opioids have been prescribed."[23] Take the drug away, and people go into withdrawal. They will do anything to stave off the symptoms. That includes going into the medicine cabinet and taking someone else's leftover prescription or going to another doctor to get a script (known as doctor shopping) or showing up at the emergency department with a complaint like abdominal pain or a back injury. Kidney stones, incredibly painful, are a common complaint for drug seekers. When they are asked to produce a urine sample, they sometimes go into the bathroom, prick their finger, and drop a little blood into their urine—a sign of a kidney stone and an indication for pain medicine. If a doctor offers Toradol or ibuprofen, the drug seeker claims to be allergic to these drugs. "What works?" the doctor inquires.

"I can't remember what they call it," the patient responds. "It starts with a *D*. Die . . . something."

"Dilaudid?" the doctor says.

"Yes, that's it!" the patient exclaims, as though the doctor has just won a game of charades. Dilaudid, of course, is a super-potent opioid.

Some people don't bother going to the ED or doctor shopping; they just buy their pills on the street. They are not hard to obtain. All you need to do is know someone who knows someone. In Hartford, oxycodone sells for one dollar a milligram. That's five dollars for a 5 mg pill or thirty dollars for a 30 mg pill.

Where do the dealers on the street get the pills? In 2013, drug companies produced 153 million kilograms of oxycodone.[24] There are a million milligrams in one kilogram. At one dollar a milligram, that's a trillion-dollar supply. No surprise, then, that pills end up on the black market. Elderly patients on a fixed income learn they can sell their pain pills for extra income. People go to a doctor's office, feign injury, and get a six-month supply of pain pills. They use some themselves and sell the rest. Also, drug companies ship to dubious suppliers who funnel massive amounts into the black market.

The nonfiction book *American Pain* by John Temple describes how two men in their twenties (one a convicted felon), who used to work construction as well as sell steroids, start a small business in which they hire doctors to write a prescription for pain medicine to almost anyone who comes through the clinic's doors. The doctors get $75 a prescription and are encouraged to see as many patients as possible. The doctors also receive $1,000 a week for the use of their DEA number (an identifier that allows health care professionals to write prescriptions for controlled substances). In no time, the clinic's waiting room and parking lot are overflowing.

Within two years, the Florida business, officially named American Pain, is bringing in $40 million a year, and a thousand other pain clinics have opened in the state. Places like Kentucky and West Virginia, which have already tightened down on opioid prescriptions, are besieged by a public health and crime crisis, as their citizens head by the vanload to Florida to return with bags of pills to use themselves and sell to locals. Two years after its doors open, American Pain, the largest pill mill in Florida, is shut down by the DEA, and the young entrepreneurs are on their way to jail, along with a few of their doctors. Most of the convictions are for charges of racketeering or illegal drug sales, but one of the entrepreneurs is convicted of first-degree murder.[25]

American Pain is a fascinating read, but by the end, I feel myself oddly wanting the young men and a couple of the doctors, despite their actions, to get leniency. I am a system-responsibility guy more than an individual-responsibility guy. I hold individuals responsible, but I also believe that systems should be held to an even higher standard. What rankles me in the end is that none of the powerful people behind the opioid epidemic, who richly profit from it, end up going to jail. Like in the financial crisis and housing collapse of 2008–2009, the common man is the one who suffers, while the perpetrators walk. The system lets these entrepreneurial knuckleheads run their business in plain sight, complete with highway billboards advertising their goods, and it does nothing until it is totally beyond control.

American Pain explains that there was little state regulation of pain clinics and that the clinic's doctors were following the "pain is what the patient says it is" credo. The clinic tried to comply with laws in its own shady way by requiring MRI scans (they made money on referrals) and urine tests (clean urine was evidently so readily available, you could buy it at area flea markets) and occasionally refusing to prescribe to clients who showed up under the influence.

In the pill mill crisis, the real bad guys are the pharmaceutical companies that make billions on OxyContin, which they know is addictive and is easily abused. They hide that fact from doctors and launch an aggressive marketing campaign to promote the drug. Surprisingly, the DEA tries to stop overprescribing and street diversions, on the one hand, while approving the manufacture of larger and larger quantities of OxyContin at the manufacturer's request, on the other hand. The book points out that earlier national epidemics involving the misuse of Quaaludes and amphetamines ended largely because the DEA cut the supply. In the OxyContin epidemic, the DEA does the exact opposite by helping Purdue Pharma flood the market with a killer drug.

What is most amazing to me in all of this is that the pill mill crisis is allowed to happen in 2009–2010, despite the publication of the 2003 exposé *Pain Killer* by *New York Times* writer Barry Meier. Meier lays out almost the same scenario of drug company promotion, widespread prescription writing, addiction, and crime, with the DEA largely going along for the ride by upping the drug limits.[26]

A report by the US congressional House Energy and Commerce Committee shows that the tiny town of Williamson, West Virginia, with a population of less than 3,200, has 20.8 million Vicodin and OxyContin pills delivered to two small pharmacies within its borders over a ten-year period.[27] All told, drug companies sell seventy-six billion pills containing opioids over the eight-year period between 2006 and 2012, with nearly half of those pills distributed by just 15 percent of the pharmacies.[28]

Between 2012 and 2013, while abuse of painkillers is becoming a national concern and the death toll is skyrocketing, the DEA still approves a production increase of more than 50 million kilograms of oxycodone.[29] Where does the DEA think the drugs will go? It must realize that many of these pills are destined for the black market. And is it any wonder that, as *60 Minutes* later reports, many high-ranking DEA officials resign to take lucrative jobs in the pharmaceutical industry?[30]

The facts are brutal: 90 percent of heroin addicts start out addicted to prescription pills.[31]

In 1996, Purdue Pharma comes out with OxyContin, a new time-released version of oxycodone. Drug users soon discover that they can crush and snort or inject the drug to receive all twelve hours' worth of pain relief at once. In 2010, Purdue Pharma reformulates OxyContin to make it hard to crush the pills into a powder and snort them. Unfortunately, the unintended side effect of making OxyContin tamper resistant is to make heroin an even more attractive alternative. Instead of a fine powder, the pills turn into clumpy goop, which makes them much harder for users to convert. Within five years, heroin deaths in the country increase fourfold.[32]

In Hartford, heroin is sold in glassine envelopes. Each envelope, which typically measures 27 millimeters, contains about 0.1 gram of powder. The powder is not all heroin, but contains cut, which could be baking soda, baby formula, sugar, aspirin, caffeine, Tylenol, Benadryl, laundry detergent, rat poison, or anything else that looks similar and increases the amount of product the dealer has to sell. The final amount of heroin in a bag is variable. Over the years, the purity level of heroin in Connecticut has risen steadily because of the abundance of white powdered heroin on the market. Even as early as 2002, the National Drug Intelligence Center was reporting that the average purity of heroin on the streets in Connecticut was 60 percent and ranging up to 95 percent.[33]

The benefit of selling high-purity powdered heroin is that it is easy to snort and, unlike cocaine, does little damage to the nasal membranes. A person who would have never considered wrapping a belt around her arm, and then injecting a needle into a vein in the crook of the elbow, now only has to snort the powder.

We get called for a seizure at 1200 Park. As we pull into the lot, red lights swirling, we are hailed by a woman standing outside the mobile phone store. She points to a battered red Buick parked outside the store. Inside, a young man is slumped out the window, shaking. On the ground outside the door, I see four empty green-and-white heroin bags labeled "Diesel" with pictures of gas pumps on them. The door is unlocked, and I open it quickly. As my partner gets out the Ambu bag, I squirt 2 milligrams of Narcan into the man's nose. We slide him onto the stretcher. His seizing has stopped, and we bag him as we get him into the back of the ambulance. Within minutes he is coming around, and I tell him what has happened to him.

"This is the first time I have ever done heroin," he says. I don't believe him, but my inclination to disbelief is stopped as he tells me his story. "I'm addicted to pain pills," he says. "I went to buy Percocets, but my dealer was out of them. I picked him up on Park Terrace. We drove around, and he told me he only had heroin. I had twenty dollars and was hoping to get a 20 mg pill; instead he sold me four bags of heroin. He told me I could snort it."

"Friend," I say, "it is way stronger."

"Evidently."

He tells me he got started using opioids on his construction job. A coworker gave him pills when his back hurt. Then when the job site closed and he lost touch with the coworker, he found himself in withdrawal, and he started buying the pills, which were expensive. His dealer told him heroin was the same as the pills, so he thought he'd try it because he was sick with withdrawal.

I hand him an emesis basin as his nausea rises. I know it will only be a matter of time before he is not only using heroin regularly but has also graduated to injecting, which increases the bang for the buck even further.

We pick up a man on lower Park Street, laid out in the road, completely unresponsive and barely breathing. A firefighter is bagging him when we arrive. The unresponsive man is tattooed all over, with thick track marks on both his arms. In the back of the ambulance, once he comes around, he tells us he had five surgeries on his legs after he was hit by a car. He was given pain pills by his doctor. "I started with Perc fives and got up to Perc twenties. Soon I needed five of those a day just to keep from feeling sick. My prescription ran out. The doc wouldn't give me more. It cost me 150 dollars a day to stay in pills. Then a friend introduced me to heroin. For thirty dollars, I get a bundle—ten bags—that lasts me for two days and does the same for me as the pills."

The economics of this is easy to understand. People addicted to prescription painkillers who buy their pills on the black market switch to heroin because heroin is cheaper and more potent. In Hartford, the going rate for oxycodone is $1 per milligram. A 30 mg oxycodone costs $30. The same person who sells oxycodone often also sells heroin. Heroin in the city goes for $4 to $5 a bag. (It can be as low as $3 a bag for regular customers.) For $30 a new user can buy, at minimum, six bags of heroin. (This is without any discount.) If the strengths were equally priced, a 30 mg oxycodone would be the equivalent of six $5 bags of heroin. But the strengths are not evenly priced. A bag of 50 percent pure heroin has twice the strength of a 30 mg oxycodone crushed to a powder and injected. For the same price as a 30 mg oxycodone, a person can buy at least six bags of heroin; each bag is two times as strong as the 30 mg oxycodone. Heroin is a better deal by a factor of at least twelve. For a user who is strapped for cash, switching to heroin is a hard deal to refuse. But it is a devil's bargain.

Kelly and Veronica

At six feet eight, I get out of the ambulance as much as I can to stretch my legs. When we are not on a call, we are posted on street corners about town in what is known as system status management, a strategy that tries to make certain that ambulances are evenly distributed across our service area to minimize response times when a 911 call comes in. Sitting in an ambulance all day can cramp you up, particularly when you have long legs like I do. I like to get out and walk around as much as I can. Sometimes I climb playground jungle gyms to stay in shape. Other times, I find a basketball court and shoot hoops or just practice spinning the basketball on my finger. I always carry a ball with me in the ambulance. I took my daughter to see the Harlem Globetrotters last winter, and she was impressed with their ball-handling abilities. My goal is to take her again next year and have my picture taken in the pregame activities the Globetrotters hold with fans. The picture will be of me expertly spinning a red, white, and blue Globetrotter basketball ball on my finger, standing next to a Globetrotter who is also spinning a similar ball on his finger.

But the main thing I do when I am out of the ambulance now is hunt for empty heroin bags. I search in areas where I have picked up overdoses in the past and places where I expect users to congregate. Users snort the powder or pour it into a cooker and then toss the bag on the ground. The city is littered with them. While some bags are blank, many of them have brands printed on them—Sweet Dreams, Killing Time, Chief. In my first month of collecting, I find fifty different brands. While I have seen bags for twenty years, I have never paid much attention to them. Four weeks before, I do three overdose calls in one day. All have the same bag at the site: Black Jack. It is printed in black and white and features the ace of hearts and king of spades. At that time our crews are doing more overdoses than anyone can remember. Spotting an envelope in the grass, I bend down and pick it up to read the brand. If there is nothing on it or if it is one I have already seen, I toss it back down. I also find numerous syringes in my travels, which I bring back to the ambulance and drop in our sharps box.

I am walking in Pope Park when I see a young woman walking toward me. She looks to be in her early twenties, a thin girl with a clear complexion and a funky punk-style hairdo: half her head is shaved, with the hair on the other side dyed purple. While I don't care for the hairstyle, she has an appealing smile as she asks, "What are you looking for?"

She has noticed my hobby. "I'm doing research," I say. "I look at the heroin bags, and I also pick up syringes so kids don't pick them up."

"Cool," she says. "What do you want to know?"

"Huh?"

"I can tell you about the brands out there. Chief is fentanyl. Have you seen that one?"

I nod that I have.

"It used to be good, but it's mainly crap now. Big Doodle is brown heroin; it's all right. They are selling just blue bags over on York Street. Those are strong, but you only get a little. Have you seen Sweet Dreams yet? I used that this morning. It's really good. It's mainly fentanyl. Sometimes when a new brand hits, it is extra strong just to get you interested."

"You're a user?" I am shocked by this thought.

"Yeah, but today's my last day using. I'm getting into rehab tomorrow. My parents are taking me to Virginia."

"Is this your first time going through rehab?"

"No, I've been twice before. I'm ready this time."

"Good for you."

"I think it will be good for me to get away from here."

"Hey, can I ask you, Did you ever use Black Jack?"

"Yeah, that was strong. My boyfriend and I could split a $4 bag and get off."

"Was that fentanyl, too?"

"Yeah. Most definitely."

"How can you tell?"

"Fentanyl has a more powerful rush, and when you throw it in the cooker, it's clear. Heroin is a more organic feeling. It itches sometimes. There hasn't been much good heroin around here for a while. It's getting to be all fentanyl."

I talk to her for half an hour. Her name is Kelly, and she is twenty-six years old. She answers every question I have. "I got into drugs when I was young," she says. "My mother was a pill head. She gave me a Percocet every time I had a headache or bad menstrual period. I liked the way it made me feel. I was at a party one night, and a guy asked me if I wanted to do some coke. It was loud at the party. I snorted the powder, and my mind exploded. What was that? I asked. It was like Percocet on steroids. Heroin, the guy told me. He had said 'dope,' and I had misheard 'coke.' Three months later I graduated from snorting heroin to injecting it. And here I am. Headed for rehab time number three."

I am sorry that she is leaving, although glad she is getting into rehab before the drugs wreck her looks and life. She is bubbly and has a great smile. She seems just like the girl next door. I never expect to see her again.

A year later we are in the ambulance in the parking lot at 1200 Park watching two people in a green Jeep shoot up heroin. The users in the car roll the window down a few inches and then toss the torn bags out. While we are watching, I notice a young woman with a pit bull on a leash walking toward us and looking at me like she might know me. When she sees me looking at her, she comes over. "Remember me?" she says.

I do. "You're Kelly, right?"

She smiles when I remember her name. She is the same girl I spoke with in the park the previous summer, except now she looks much worse. Her hair under her New York Yankees baseball cap is dirty and unkempt. Her face and arms are scabbed with insect bites. She still has a nice smile, but she looks like she hasn't slept in days.

"Last I saw you, you were headed to rehab in, was it in Virginia?"

"I never made it," she says. "My boyfriend, Tom, showed up and talked me out of it."

"That's too bad. Are you still living with your parents?"

"No, I'm homeless."

"Oh, no, that must be rough."

She shrugs. "Hey, can you look at my foot for me? I have an ulcer that isn't healing."

"Sure," I say. She unrolls a dirty sock to reveal a few weeping ulcers. They are not from needle marks but are more like dirty blisters that aren't healing.

"You don't have any ointment, do you?"

"No, but I can get you some."

She tells me she's been living under the highway. We have noticed a lot of people walking back that way in recent weeks. Kelly says there are about fifteen of them living there, mostly all in their twenties or early thirties. The police don't bother them there, but the bugs can be bad, and with her anxiety, she is picking at the bites all the time. I ask her about the dog. Diamond, she calls her. Diamond is very loyal and protective. I can see how that would come in handy for a young single woman of slight build living on the streets. She does point out to me her boyfriend, who is across the parking lot, going through garbage receptacles looking for bottles or food. I ask her what bags are out there, and she tells me Rolex is the best—it is all fentanyl. It has a nice rush, although not as good as when it first came out last week.

Our conversation is interrupted when we get a 911 call for a motor vehicle crash on Mohegan Drive. After that, I go to a CVS Pharmacy and do some shopping.

When we return to 1200 Park, Kelly sits with her pit bull outside the market. There is a small dish of water for the dog and a bag of several empty plastic bottles she will no doubt redeem. She and the dog look sad. I hand her a plastic bag from CVS. Inside are cortisone cream for her bites, some protein bars, a bottle of water, a can of food for the dog, and a five-dollar bill.

I thought long and hard about the five-dollar bill and discussed it with my new partner Bryan Sabin. Bryan is in his late forties. He worked for many years as a community organizer and is our union rep. From a political point of view, he is as liberal a person as works at our company, in a field otherwise dominated by conservatives. Maybe she will use it for food, but there is a good chance she will use it for heroin, we agree. I have read recently that the pope says it is okay to give money to the homeless. The pope says it doesn't matter what they are going to use it for. Bryan agrees that charity shouldn't come with strings attached. Five dollars will brighten her day and let her spend less time sitting by the market door hoping that people will give her their spare change.

Later I look up the article about the pope. He says that when you give a poor person money and he spends it on wine, you should not think that wrong. If "a glass of wine is the only happiness he has in life, that's OK." What is important, the pope says, is the manner of giving: "Tossing money and not looking in their eyes is not a Christian way." When giving charity, one should do it "by looking them in the eyes and touching their hands."[1]

Kelly gives me a big smile when I hand her the bag and mention there is food for Diamond inside and some protein bars for her along with the ointment. I don't say anything about the five-dollar bill, but I know she sees it when she opens the bag. She thanks me, but before I can talk with her more, we get another 911 call. When we turn out of the shopping center parking lot, our lights and sirens on, I look back to see if she is still sitting there, but now she is up and on the move, walking over in the direction where her boyfriend is still going through trash cans looking for empty bottles to recycle at a nickel a pop.

Our run gets canceled before we arrive at the scene, and when we swing back, I see her scurrying up Park Street by herself (no boyfriend and no dog). She looks like a little girl off to see Santa Claus.

As time goes by, I start to make friends with more and more of the users in Hartford. Some of them I meet on 911 calls; others I just see on the street. On hot days, I bring a cooler of water bottles packed in ice that I hand out to people who look hot. I also carry oranges and apples. You look hungry, I'll say, as I hand them an orange and a dollar bill. We station the ambulance across from Pope Park, and sometimes users will stop by and talk. Some will ask for medical advice about their abscesses, and I'll direct them to the ED or local clinics. If they have open wounds that are dirty, I give them water, antibiotic ointment, and fresh bandages I get for a dollar a package at the dollar store. Keep it clean, I say, and go to the clinic.

In return for water, fruit, and a few dollar bills, I get to hear their stories. I could spend fifteen dollars to go to the movies, but I'd rather pass that money out on Hartford's streets and listen to far truer stories, and often more moving stories, than I would see on the big screen.

Veronica is one of my favorites. The first time I pick up Veronica is on Hungerford Street. We are called for an unresponsive person, but instead we find a small woman with a limp who is staggering down the sidewalk. She is half on the nod and covered with leaves. I ask her if she is okay as we walk up. She just mumbles and tries to keep walking. We stand in front of her, and at twice her size, we are hard for her to ignore. We were called, we explain, so we have to see if she is okay at least.

"I'm fine," she says. "I just want to go home."

"Why are you covered with leaves?" I ask.

She wipes tears from her eyes. "The kids robbed me and threw me in the bushes. It happens all the time. They like having their fun with me."

At least she seems to have managed to buy and use some heroin before they accosted her. Her pupils are pinpoint, and she has a weakness in her knees while standing. Perhaps the kids were warned by the block enforcer not to rob her until she had contributed her few crumpled dollars to the day's take.

"You don't hurt anywhere?"

"No, I just want to go home."

She is under the influence, but she is breathing fine and knows where she is when asked. She lets Jerry do a head-to-toe survey of her, and he finds nothing significant. We can't talk her into going to the hospital, but we do walk her the two blocks home to her building, where a neighbor who sees her walking with us agrees to look after her. She tells us she has Narcan in her apartment.

After that day, whenever I see Veronica on the street, I have Jerry pull the ambulance to the curb and I call out, "Hey, Veronica, how are you?" She comes to the ambulance window and we chat. I usually give her an orange and maybe a couple bucks to get something to eat. She loves slices of pizza.

Through our conversations, I gradually learn about her life. She is thirty-eight. When she was a young girl she wanted to be a dancer, but her bones were too brittle to stand up to the stress. She once went to New York to see *Swan Lake* on Broadway, and she has ice-skated at Rockefeller Center. She turned to pain pills and then heroin for her bone pain and for other health reasons, which she does not elaborate on. She says she stays away from white heroin because she is afraid of overdosing on fentanyl, which has already happened to her twice, when she woke up looking at paramedics. She snorts and does not inject, as she is afraid of needles, despite the colorful butterfly tattoo I can see on her forearm. She stays away from the brands Chief, KD, and Fastrack. She makes certain to keep Narcan in her apartment and tries not to use alone, although she admits she often does.

We are at the substance abuse rehab hospital, waiting for a nurse to let us into the locked unit to take out a patient with low oxygen saturation, when I see Veronica come out of the entrance elevator and walk up to the admission desk. She is very pale and moves like every bone and muscle in her body is aching.

"Veronica," I call over to her. "How are you doing?" She looks about the room trying to locate the familiar voice. She likely isn't expecting to be recognized here. When she sees me, she forces a smile and nods recognition. "Glad to see you," I say. "This is your time. You can do it." She looks down at her feet, her face flushing. I am not certain if she is pleased I said hi or if I embarrassed her.

That is the last I see of her for many months. And then, just before Christmas, I spot her walking alone on Park Street early in the morning. We pull over, and I call out her name. She comes over, her head barely up to the window. When I ask her where she has been, she tells me she has been staying with her sister in Woodbury, but then she slipped up. Now she is back in Hartford. I tell her that I am proud of her for the months she's been clean and that she shouldn't be discouraged. Relapse is a part of recovery for many. She did it once; she can do it again. Next time will be the charm.

"Thank you," she says.

I reach in my pocket and take out a Dunkin' Donuts gift card. I always keep a few on me to give to homeless people. "Merry Christmas," I say, then add, "It's only for five dollars."

Her face softens, and she gives me a huge smile. She takes it with one hand, and with the other, she reaches for my hand and gives it a squeeze. "Merry Christmas," she says.

I watch her hobble down the street and wonder what her Christmas will be like, if she will be spending it with family and friends or if she will celebrate it by snorting a bag of heroin alone in her apartment. I wish I had given her a few bucks to go with the card or maybe the orange I had with me.

I try to follow the users I encounter and see how they are progressing with their lives. Some I see regularly on Park Street; others disappear. I don't know if they die or if they recover and are living productive lives or if they are just using on the streets of another city. I can't see the future, but every day that people are still alive should be counted as a small victory for them, even if they fail in the end.

I still see Veronica around the neighborhood, and sometimes we talk. She lost her apartment and now stays here and there, sometimes living outside, sometimes crashing with friends and acquaintances. She has graduated to injecting. Her hands are already scarred, and I can even see needle marks in her neck. I see her one morning on Park Street. It is a bitterly cold morning. She is with three guys wearing hoodies, whom I always see in front of the same shuttered store. She does a wobbly dance for them, prancing around, turning circles, and waving a scarf in the air. She laughs and they laugh too. They seem to think her dancing is funny, like she is their court jester. They motion for her to dance more, and she responds, flapping her arms like a butterfly. I have a brief vision of her then, just flying away, rising above Park Street and soaring on a kind wind to a better place. The vision fades, and all I see are the men laughing as she stumbles.

My partner asks if I want him to stop so I can say hi to her, but I tell him to keep driving.

Opioid Conference

When I work for Governor Weicker from 1991 to 1995, I have an office in the Public Health Department that looks out on Washington Street, where I can see ambulances racing past toward Hartford Hospital, where I see the Life Star helicopter land on the rooftop. I wear a coat and tie, make a decent salary, and have an American flag lapel pin, but I feel the sirens calling to me.

When I was younger and realized I would never be good enough to play right field for the Boston Red Sox, my second choice was to follow in the footsteps of John F. Kennedy and become president. I am totally committed to the mantra of "Ask not what your country can do for you, but what you can do for your country." I first go to work for Weicker in 1976 as an unpaid intern in a Washington, DC, semester program offered by my high school. I ask to work for him not only because he is the junior senator from Connecticut but also because I watched him on the Senate Watergate committee, where, as a Republican, he stood up to his own party when it became apparent to him that President Richard Nixon had committed criminal wrongdoing. I remember being riveted when Weicker proclaimed, "Let me make it clear, because I've got to have my partisan moment. Republicans do not cover up.

Republicans do not go ahead and threaten. Republicans do not commit illegal acts, and God knows Republicans don't view their fellow Americans as enemies to be harassed, but rather I can assure you that Republicans and those that I serve with look upon every American as a human being to be loved and won."[1] To me the moment is every bit as heroic as a ballplayer making a game-saving diving catch in the outfield.

I take a year off before starting college and work for Weicker, and then later I work part-time and summers for him during college. While in school I fall under the spell of the great American writers Ernest Hemingway, John Steinbeck, and Jack Kerouac. I realize I am not always the most outgoing person and am unlikely to run for even town office, much less president, so I decide I want to be a writer. My life follows a pattern of working odd jobs and struggling to write and then coming back to work for Weicker. But Weicker is beaten in his reelection attempt in 1988. His independence costs him dearly. Many Republicans vote for his Democratic opponent, Joe Lieberman, who runs to the right of Weicker, even publicly embracing conservative commentator William F. Buckley.

I suddenly find myself out of work at thirty and uncertain what to do. I enjoyed the TV show *Emergency* when I was young, and so unable to play for the Red Sox or become president, I decide to try to become an EMT and find glory under the lights and siren. When Weicker decides to run for governor, I am his issues manager, while still working one night a week on the ambulance. Once he becomes governor, I continue to ride the ambulance and even go to paramedic school at night, while writing speeches for him during the day and serving as the executive assistant to the commissioner in the state health department. While I admire Weicker, I do not like sitting behind a desk. Instead of watching city activity through a glass window, I want to be out there on the streets below. When his term ends, and he does not run for reelection, my plan is to work full-time as a 911 paramedic and use my government experience to help improve the emergency health care system from my firsthand observations.

I do just that. The day Weicker leaves office is my first day as a paramedic in Hartford. For twenty-five years, I bring my field experience to the table as I work on improving stroke, heart attack, and trauma systems. I never regret that decision. I feel as though I have found my place in the world. I regularly work sixty to seventy hours a week, making a good income with all the overtime, and still find time to attend committee meetings and write two books and a blog about being a paramedic. In 2008, I trade in my overtime hours for a part-time job as the EMS coordinator at UConn John Dempsey Hospital.

In the same week that I treat a cheerleader who overdosed and crashed her car, I read another paramedic's run form describing finding a father doing CPR on his overdosed daughter. The narrative is sparse, but chilling:

> Upon arrival found a 24 Y/O female unresponsive lying on the floor of her bedroom with her father performing CPR on her. He states that he last saw her alive an hour ago and then found her on the floor unconscious before calling 911. He states she has a history of heroin abuse and there is a used needle lying next to her. She is unresponsive, with no palpable pulse and she is apneic.

I have done similar calls and know other medics who have also. The rash of overdoses we are seeing in the field is not just the result of a bad batch of heroin, but rather overdose is becoming the norm. Young people are dying all around us without anybody paying much attention.

On a day when I do three overdose runs, all for the same brand of heroin, Black Jack, I start paying more attention to the heroin bags. My eyes are opened. I start noticing that the bags are as plentiful on the ground as cigarette butts. In following the bags, I soon start finding the users, and a new world, which has been all around me, opens up. I begin talking to my patients about their drug use, and as I begin to see them as normal people whose lives were upended by a chance injury or encounter, I become obsessed with learning as much as I can about the opioid epidemic.

Through a friend in the FBI, who rides with me in the city one day as an observer, I am introduced to Kelsey Opozda, a health policy analyst for New England HIDTA (High Intensity Drug Trafficking Area). She tells me about an upcoming state conference on the opioid epidemic as well as a working group that meets once a month in Hartford to discuss issues related to the crisis. The conference is booked up, but I am able to plead my way on to the list. I have to take a day off from the ambulance to go, but it is worth it. There are not many people from EMS here. The one I do recognize is Raffaella "Ralf" Coler, who is the head of the state EMS office. She taught my EMT-Intermediate class thirty years ago, and we have been friends ever since. She is excited to see me and asks what I am doing there. "This is where EMS should be," I say, realizing it perhaps for the first time. This is where we have the potential to make a big difference, I think, if we can only figure out how.

Ralf and I sit at a table with some interesting people, including Sarah Howroyd and Chief Marc Montminy of the Manchester Police Department. Manchester is a small city of fifty-eight thousand located east of the Connecticut River. Sarah is a social worker and an ex-user who, working with the police chief, has started a program called the HOPE (Heroin/Opioid Prevention and Education) Initiative, through which the police help get users into treatment instead of jail. HOPE also hosts events to train people in naloxone use, connect people with recovery resources, and teach ways to prevent opioid use. Marc is a police chief who realized his department couldn't arrest its way out of the crisis. The two of them are changing the way police departments across the state are handling people who use opioids.

Also seated at the table is Ed Leahy, who works for Adapt Pharma, a company that is marketing a new 4 mg intranasal Narcan spray, which at this time has not yet been approved in Connecticut for EMS. Ralf and I have a heated discussion with Ed about the dose, which we think is way too high to give EMS providers, who can use an Ambu bag to breathe for patients while waiting for a more reasonable dose to work. The goal is not to knock all the opioids out of their system and so throw them into withdrawal; it is simply to restore their breathing. In an ideal situation, they won't even know they have gotten naloxone. The 4 mg intranasal dose is equivalent to 2 milligrams of intramuscular Narcan, given its lower bioavailability. A 0.4 mg dose is a more reasonable starting place unless the patient is completely apneic (not breathing). I do agree with Ed that the Adapt device is simple to use. Unlike the current atomizer setup, in which a drug vial is inserted into a syringe and then an atomizer is screwed onto the syringe, this device requires no assembly. It is a true nasal spray: you simply insert the nozzle in a patient's nostril and push. The 4 milligrams are contained in only 0.1 cubic centimeter of fluid, whereas the atomizer device uses 2 milligrams in 2 cubic centimeters, which is so much fluid that much of the Narcan is either lost down the throat or else comes back out of the nostril. Of the 2 milligrams, the patient may be getting only 0.2 to 0.4 milligram, which still, in most cases, is enough to restore breathing. I do see how the simple 4 mg device would be great for laypeople or a responder on call alone.

While many laypeople are already using the device thanks to Connecticut's community naloxone laws, other organizations will not carry it because it is not approved for EMS. Our current state protocol restricts EMS to giving a maximum of 2 milligrams in an initial dose. In time, I help Ed get the new 4 mg dose approved in Connecticut by inviting him to our regional medical advisory council, where he presents on the device. With the region's

approval, the issue goes to the state board, where it is also ac-
cepted. Once approved for state protocol, the Hartford police and
fire department will adopt it, and I will no longer show up on the
scene to find police officers directing traffic around a car with an
unresponsive driver or come upon firefighters fumbling with the
atomizer setup. Instead, they are able to deliver the medicine
promptly and resuscitate the patient sooner, possibly saving a life
by restarting breathing. Unfortunately, the drawback is that, on
numerous occasions, I arrive to find an agitated patient being
held down or a patient vomits on me the moment I arrive because
the higher dose put that person into full-scale withdrawal.

The conference fascinates me. I learn about the action plan of the
Connecticut Opioid Response Initiative, commissioned by Governor Dannel P. Malloy, which includes six strategies to fight the
epidemic:

1. Increase access to treatment, consistent with national
   guidelines, with methadone and buprenorphine.
2. Reduce overdose risk, especially among those individuals
   at highest risk.
3. Increase adherence to opioid prescribing guidelines among
   providers, especially those providing prescriptions associated with an increased risk of overdose and death.
4. Increase access to and track use of naloxone.
5. Increase data sharing across relevant agencies and organizations to monitor and facilitate responses, including rapid
   responses to "outbreaks" of overdoses and other opioid-
   related events (e.g., outbreaks of HIV or hepatitis C virus).
6. Increase community understanding of the scale of opioid
   use disorder, the nature of the disorder, and the most
   effective evidence-based responses to promote treatment
   uptake and decrease stigma.[2]

I hear about a concept called harm reduction from Mark Jenkins of the Greater Hartford Harm Reduction Coalition. I later learn that Mark grew up in Hartford's north end and, after getting out of the army, fought his own drug and alcohol use for ten years before becoming a volunteer to help others fight their addictions. In time, harm reduction becomes his "ministry."

When it is Mark's turn to present, he moves slowly up to the podium, with all eyes upon him, and I can sense he is known to most all in the room. Some love him and others, I sense, see him as a pain in the ass. He has a mischievous smile that warms the room no matter what anyone thinks of him. If only he had a long white beard, he could be Santa Claus.

Mark starts by defining harm reduction. He quotes a friend of the movement. "We are," he says, "a close-knit family of dreamers, radicals, and outsiders tempering anger with hope, fighting stigma and marginalization with love."

Those words get my attention.

"We are in the midst of an epidemic unlike anything we engaged or have had to deal with in our generation," Mark declares, and I can clearly imagine him not as a speaker in front of our room but as a minister preaching to a packed church on Sunday:

> The loss of life is staggering, and although a lot of work has been done and continues to be done, many of us haven't changed the method of how that work gets done. We still have this cookie-cutter thing going on, and we squeeze people into this cookie-cutter realm of having to recover, yet we still know only a small portion of the people that we engage are really seeking recovery. If there's some 2.2 million people that we engage, there are 40 million people using. Shouldn't we begin to try to see how we are going to engage all of these people over there before they get over here? How do we do that?
>
> Harm reduction acknowledges that people use drugs along the continuum just like the stages of change. We design and promote

programs to address a public health nightmare. Yet we're seen, for the most part, as enablers. Harm reduction has existed for many, many years, and for many years, we are considered the bastard stepchild of prevention. You knew we were there, but we were ignored because they didn't want to mess with us, because when you open the door, they don't go away. They see me and it's, oh God, here he comes again. I have one promise for you. When people stop dying, I'll stop coming. When people stop dying, I'll stop poking holes in a lot of the great work that we're doing because in many cases it's just not enough; it's because that part that becomes enough is what offends our morals.

We have to understand why people use drugs. It's because they work; they work for whatever it is they need them to work for until they no longer work. When they find themselves in a position where they no longer work, it is usually somewhere dark, and they are by themselves, and everyone can sometimes become the enemy.

As I listen to his words, I am struck, as I always am, by someone with the courage to speak inconvenient truths. He talks about needle exchange and safe-injection sites. He speaks of the basic humanity that people must recognize in each other. His gist is that if you treat users like people, keep up a conversation with them, then when they are ready, you can bring them in from the cold; and if they are never ready, you can at least help keep them alive, keep them a part of the community, and prevent the harm they may do to themselves and others. "Let's keep people alive," Mark says, "so that they can be around to make the decision that if recovery is something they want, we can point them in that direction. We all know that dead people don't make good decisions."

He receives a rousing ovation, and even those whose well-meaning programs he has indirectly criticized clap for him in earnest. You have to appreciate his authenticity. I think to myself, this is a man I want to get to know and learn from.

I have already started furiously making notes. I think maybe EMS can help in this harm reduction fight, as well as in other areas. We have so far, aside from treatment and transport, been on the sidelines of the opioid war, but we could clearly become key players. In a few years, the notes and conversations germinating this day will come to life on a scale I could not have imagined.

During a break, I talk with Kelsey and her partner Robert Lawlor about an idea for an early warning system, where EMTs call in to a central location after each overdose. If they find a bag on the scene, they report it. This way, if a new brand hits the streets that is especially potent, it can be identified quickly. Public safety can work to get the brand off the street, and harm reduction workers can alert users to be careful. Kelsey and her partner like the idea, although there are many challenges to work out.

I have much to process by the time the day is over. From the programs and ideas to the sheer emotion of the opioid crisis, I know this is an area I want to become involved with. To be a successful contributor, EMS will first need to be educated about addiction and understand that it is not a character flaw but rather a disease, and those who fall victim to the disease don't do so as a result of free will.

Besides Mark Jenkins, the one other speaker at the conference whom I would most want my fellow first responders to hear is the father of a boy who died of an overdose. With the help of a slideshow, the father tells the story of a loving family and a son's struggles—in and out of rehab, doing well then relapsing—until the family finally receives the dreaded phone call informing them that their son is dead.

The father's words stick with me: "Sometimes there is not enough love in the world to beat this. Heroin was simply too strong for my son."

Harm Reduction

A dispatch directs us to West Hartford, Hartford's wealthy cousin. A parent can't wake up a son. I am hoping it is not another cardiac arrest. We charge up the stairs. In the bedroom, we find a father trying to shake the young man, who lies in bed, breathing shallowly but not responding. His pupils are pinpoint. "Any history of opioid use?" I ask the father, as I take out the naloxone and give his son two squirts up the nose and my partner gets the Ambu bag out to assist his breathing.

"He's been clean for six months," the man says. "He doesn't use anymore."

"Well, it looks like he had a relapse."

Already I can see his respiratory rate picking up. In another moment he opens his eyes and looks around. He sees his father. "I'm sorry," he says.

"I thought you gave this up. We had a deal."

"I'm sorry," he says again.

"I can't believe this," the father says. "After all that rehab."

I ease myself between them and ask the father if I can talk to him in the hallway. "Don't be too hard on him," I say once we are alone. "It is a difficult battle. Relapse is expected."

He shakes his head, still unbelieving about what has occurred.

"You should have naloxone in the house," I say. "Do you know where to get it?"

"But he doesn't use anymore. He's clean."

"That doesn't matter. Relapse can always happen. You should keep some in the medicine cabinet just in case. It could save his life."

I tell him he can get naloxone at the nearest pharmacy, or his doctor can also prescribe it for him. I wish then that I had a pamphlet of some kind I could give the man. I show him how easy it is to assemble the intranasal naloxone. Two squirts up the nose, one in each nostril, and then call 911. I am surprised that he does not already know this. I learn that the rehab the son attended was out of state and that the counselors had told him that, after thirty days in their facility, his son was now in good shape, clean and with a positive attitude. This is his son's only relapse.

Later, I will hear the story of Waterbury fire captain Gary LeBlanc's first experience taking his son to rehab. He and his wife met another set of parents there whose son was in rehab for the sixth time. LeBlanc thought, *that won't be my son. One time will be the charm.* Today, six rehabs later, Gary's son has not used going on nine months. When Gary is at an overdose scene, he gives his phone number to parents and tells them they can call him anytime. He also has a handwritten list of resources he gives to them.

EMS ought to have printed material, I think, something we can leave with the family that both says addiction is a disease, not a character defect, and offers the family avenues to help. I remember that, in my briefcase, I have a pamphlet Mark Jenkins passed out at the conference. When we get down to the ambulance, I give one to the father, and I make a note about developing a special EMS handout as something to add to my list of things to do.

The son cries on the way to the hospital. He broke his leg playing football, he tells me. That started his journey. He says that he wasn't intending to use again after rehab, but he ran into the guy who used to sell to him. He thought he could use just once because he was depressed about a relationship.

"You can't use the same amount you used to," I say. "Your tolerance is down."

He just shakes his head. "My father is so upset," he says. "I hate putting him through any more of this. I think he's starting to hate me."

"No, you're his son," I say. "I'm sure he wants the best for you."

It occurs to me then that most of the users I revive with naloxone, if they admit to using drugs, are remorseful and self-hating. I don't believe I have the language yet to know what to say, how to make him feel better about himself and, at the same time, to get through to him that this is a real opportunity for change. Who am I to tell him what to do?

Hospitals in Connecticut are experimenting with recovery coaches.[1] Recovery coaches are former users who meet overdose victims at the ED and offer help. Because coaches have been through it themselves and made it through to the other side, users may be more inclined listen to them and heed their advice. The coaches can help people navigate the difficult recovery path and serve as a source of hope. Typically, once an overdose patient is brought to the ED and expresses a willingness to talk with a coach, the coach is then called to come in to the ED. I imagine a day when, on the way to the hospital with an overdose patient, the ambulance crew calls in an opioid alert, indicating that someone who needs immediate counseling is soon to arrive. The ED can then page the on-call recovery coach, in the same manner that EMS now calls in stroke, heart attack, and trauma alerts. By being in the ED ready to treat a patient as soon as he is brought through the doors, the on-call neurologist, cardiac interventionalist, or trauma surgeon may save that person's life. Likewise, a recovery coach could do the same if she is able to reach the user and get him on the pathway to recovery, instead of the hospital discharging him back to Park Street. Most of my EMS colleagues and I cannot serve as recovery coaches, not having been through opioid recovery ourselves, but we can share information, show empathy, and advocate for our patients.

Saint Francis Hospital starts a new program where users who meet certain criteria can get Suboxone right in the ED. Suboxone, a milder opioid than heroin, both eases their withdrawal symptoms and dampens their cravings. Users in the Suboxone program are then given a "warm handoff" to a treatment program by getting a ride right to the program's doors. If patients express even the slightest interest in getting on Suboxone, I make certain to take them to Saint Francis.

One day, as I am walking through a parking lot on Albany Avenue, stretching my legs and looking for heroin bags, my eye is caught by an odd-looking bunch of papers. It turns out to be a sixteen-page photocopied, folded, and stapled comic book called *Lil' Dope Fiend Overdose Prevention Guide*. It is the craziest comic book I have ever seen. It teaches readers how to use Narcan and do rescue breathing and when to call 911. It seems to have been put together by a drug user for other drug users, and it is hysterically funny, in addition to being quite accurate. To test if someone needs resuscitation, the book teaches readers to watch the user's breathing. If the overdosed user is not breathing or has shallow breathing, readers are advised to rub their knuckles on the other person's sternum—an EMS trick. Then, if the person is still not responding, readers are instructed to say, "I'm going to Narcan you! I'm taking all your dope!"—which is definitely not an EMS-sanctioned trick. If neither of these measures elicits a response, the user definitely needs Narcan. Readers are told to call 911.

We are driving through the lot at 1200 Park looking for Kelly, when I see a familiar round-faced man sitting on the back of an open van. There is a giant sharps box on the ground next to him. He breaks into a big smile as we drive up. It's Mark Jenkins, the harm reduction man. Once users see him out there, word spreads, and people come from under the highway overpass, and cars pull up and users step out. It is a Sunday, and the local needle exchange van operates only Monday through Friday. Many have already run out of their supply of fresh needles, so this is a welcome event. The users hand over their old needles, counting them out as they drop them in the sharps box, and Mark hands them new syringes, ten to a package. I am amazed at the number of syringes some of the users pull out of their backpacks. One of the advantages of needle exchange is that users pick up used needles, knowing they can exchange them for new ones. They use some of the new needles themselves and sell some to other users for a dollar apiece.

Mark also hands out clean tourniquets, bottle-cap cookers, saline bullets (vials of sterile solution to mix with heroin), alcohol wipes, and little bits of cotton. Users dump their heroin in the bottle cap, squirt in saline water, stir it until it dissolves, often heat the mixture to sterilize it, and then draw it up through the cotton ball, which serves to filter out impurities.

Mark has another product for them today: fentanyl test strips. "Stick the strip in your cooker," Mark says. "If one line turns red, there is fentanyl present; two lines, it's negative. You can choose not to use or, if you do, do a test shot. Do two bags instead of five. Have someone with you."

When I mention to Mark the comic book I found, he says he is familiar with it. In fact, he is likely where it came from, as it is one of his most popular handouts. He often puts copies of it in the Narcan kits he hands out. He provides a user with a quick training and then hands him a red bag containing two naloxone vials, two 1 cc syringes, two needles, alcohol prep pads, latex gloves, a cooker, and some educational pamphlets.

Mark tells me he has also been collecting heroin bags across the city. At present, nearly 90 percent of the city's bags have fentanyl in them. "It's about informed choices," Mark says. "They can choose to avoid the fentanyl, or much more likely, if they use it, they at least know it's there, and they can take steps to stay safe, having someone there with them, having naloxone available, using less than they normally would."

The test strips were developed to test urine for the presence of fentanyl, but they work just as well when the drug is mixed with water. After a user has mixed his drug in his cooker and drawn up his shot, he is instructed to add a little water to the cooker. He dips the test strip in the water, then sets it on the cooker and waits thirty seconds for the results. One red line indicates fentanyl; two lines mean none. If a person snorts instead of injects, she can tap the contents out of the heroin bag, add a little water to the residue in the emptied bag, and then dip the strip.

In 2017, a pilot study is done in San Francisco that shows a prevalence of fentanyl in the city's heroin supply. Over half the users report testing their supply before using, with many subsequently using harm reduction strategies. Over half also share their findings with others in the community. The strips not only help inform users of what they're putting into their bodies, but they also provide another chance for valuable dialogue between users and harm reduction workers.[2]

"God bless," a user says to Mark after getting his test strips.

"If you ever need clean needles or help, here's my number." Mark hands him his card. He will get up in the middle of the night to help someone. It may be just to give him clean needles to help avoid infections like HIV or hepatitis C, or it could be the moment of human contact when a user becomes ready to come in from the cold. Mark is there to help him along the way, getting him into a program or other safe harbor. "Be safe, brother," Mark says.

Mark gives me some fentanyl test strips and more of his cards that I can pass on to users. "Any time of day or night, I'll meet them," he says.

We invite Mark to speak at several of the regional EMS seminars that Ralf Coler, Rich Kamin (the state EMS medical director), and I put together to teach EMS workers about the epidemic. The speakers cover everything from the epidemic's origins to harm reduction. Kelsey Opozda and Robert Lawlor talk about fentanyl and other drug trends in Connecticut. Sarah Howroyd talks about her experiences as a user and now director of the HOPE (Heroin/Opioid Prevention and Education) Initiative. Other speakers cover the origins of the epidemic and the science of addiction. When Mark speaks to the audience about harm reduction, many are stunned to hear someone advocating giving drug users the tools of their trade, not just clean needles and sterile cookers but crack-safe inhalation kits, which include mouthpieces to prevent users from burning their throat.

While some of the medics are shocked by what they are hearing, they also have the ability to recognize authenticity. This isn't some academic kook talking to them but a man from the streets who knows what he is talking about. By the end of his presentation, he has changed many minds.

Mark Jenkins was born on Kent Street in Hartford's north end. He was raised on the same streets he walks today, and those streets led him to drugs as a young man. He smoked marijuana and drank alcohol, but above all, he favored cocaine. When he joined the US Air Force, he was stationed in the Pacific Northwest, where he used crystal methamphetamine. He married, had a child, and lost both wife and child to his drug use.

Once back east he tried heroin for the first time, on the advice of a fellow stimulant user who said it would mellow him out. He would, in his words, "Scarface" bags, snorting the powder quickly into his nose; and while he did get mellowed out, every time he used, he ended up vomiting. That kept him from getting too deeply into it.

Over the course of eleven years, Mark was in rehab seventeen times. He says he was fine in rehab and could recite all the right answers to the questions put to him. He knew what drugs did and how you could avoid drugs, but once he got out of each program, the "obsession and compulsion" was too great. Back on the street, he still didn't know how to apply that knowledge: "Give me a fifty-dollar bill, and that was all it took to get me back on the road to self-destruction."

In the end he was able to break the cycle only through a combination of fortuitous events and friendships. He was sick and tired of the seemingly endless cycle of his life: "I was either going to kill someone, or I was going to get killed." As a young man, Mark was into music; he was a deejay who occasionally had his spinning aired on the radio. He got a turntable and a mixer and started working again. One night, after deejaying at a sober dance, he met an outreach worker he knew who was also an ex-user. The man looked at him and said, "you are one of the winners."

"I didn't believe it myself," Mark says, "but if he believed it, I thought maybe it was possible." Mark went to school for general studies and realized he still had a couple of firing brain cells. Perhaps the most important factor in his survival was the people he started hanging out with. They were a group of AIDS outreach workers who had helped him get into treatment. He felt safe with them. He ended up volunteering, answering phones. That led to a part-time job, and then another part-time job. He worked at the local Veterans Administration center, helping fellow veterans. To support himself he also drove limos and continued to develop his deejay business. A position with AIDS Project Hartford opened up, for doing outreach to hard-to-reach populations, and he got the position.

He found himself doing work that was comfortable for him. "Like a pair of shoes," he says, "it fit." In the coming years, he met a number of people who influenced his life. Mark Kinzley, Dennis Knapp, and Tony Gibbons introduced him to harm reduction. "I was a hard-core twelve-stepper. I felt that if people wanted what I had, they had to do what I did." But these new friends taught Mark another way. Harm reduction is about acknowledging people for who they are, treating them with empathy instead of just sympathy, and doing what is best to keep them alive until they are ready. And if they are never ready for rehab, harm reduction is about keeping them alive in the state they are in. Mark, Tony, Dennis, and others were giving out naloxone to users long before it was legal. They were disciples of a man named Dan Bigg, of the Chicago Recovery Alliance, whom Mark refers to as the godfather of layman naloxone. It wasn't about legal right or wrong; it was about saving people's lives. To Mark, this new work felt like what he should be doing.

On the wall of Mark's office, there are dozens of pictures of people whom he has met along the way, not all of them still with us. But he points to each of them with love and talks about what each of them taught him. The names likely mean nothing to most of us, but to those involved in harm reduction, and those who have benefited from the presence and grace of these people, they are a hall of fame of kindness and belief in the humanity of every soul, no matter how hard people have fallen or the hardships that befell them. These men and women, Mark's teachers and mentors, look down proudly on the work he is continuing. The picture of Mark and Tony is poster size. It shows the two men smiling. Tony, Mark tells me, overdosed and died on the job. Many of the people like Tony, who helped Mark along his path, relapsed themselves and died. Even Dan Bigg, the man who popularized needle exchange and naloxone distribution to users and their families, dies of a fentanyl overdose in August 2018.[3] In obituaries, he is remembered as a man who "saved tens of thousands of lives" and a man who "did not give two fucks about what was allowed. He only cared about what was right."[4] Today, Dan Bigg and Tony Gibbons and many others are gone from the earth, but their love and their work and their lessons live on in Mark.

In 2010, Mark went to a national harm reduction conference in Austin, Texas. There, he met more future friends, people who were doing the same work he was. While in Connecticut, outreach was losing favor—the work was moving from the streets to offices—Mark recommitted to staying in the field. When AIDS Project Hartford merged with another organization, Mark lost his job. But he didn't stop doing the work. Mark harnessed the resentment he felt on being bypassed. In March 2014, he founded the Greater Hartford Harm Reduction Coalition. *Who better to do the work than me?* he thought. He was invested in his community, and when running the show, he could do what he thought was needed without having to run it through a bureaucracy. He walked away from his deejay business, which had become successful, and devoted himself to the work of harm reduction. "People were falling through the cracks and not getting the basic services to remediate their drug use," he says. He wouldn't let that happen.

Tony and Mark used to tell him, "Always take care of yourself; don't let the work consume you." But for Mark, who seems tireless in his ministry, "it's not work; it's a way to live with passion."

I have walked this earth for sixty years and can count on my fingers the number of people I have met who truly impress me. Mark is one of them. "Call me at any hour," he says to a user, "and I'll get you help." His word is good.

When I respond to overdose calls and talk to users, I might direct them to Mark. It's amazing how many people know him. A bystander, who gave Narcan to a man who minutes before had overdosed and was not breathing, says to me, "Oh, yeah, Mark's the one who gave me that Narcan. He trained all of us."

I think if we in EMS spoke Mark's harm reduction language, and showed his compassion, we could make a difference far beyond our routine treat and transport. There is a role for EMS beyond simply providing naloxone to people in overdose. Those who are most at risk of fatal overdose are those with a prior non-fatal overdose. These are the people whom EMS responders help. We are in the perfect place to make an intervention. Maybe we can be harm reductionists like Mark and join his army, I think. And with the growing fentanyl danger out there, he is going to need the numbers.

Fentanyl

On February 2, 1991, according to an article in the *Hartford Courant*, a man collapses dead in his apartment after shooting up heroin in a brick public housing project known as Stowe Village in Hartford's north end.[1] The brand he uses is called "Tango and Cash," named after the undercover-cop buddy movie starring Sylvester Stallone and Kurt Russell. Before the weekend is over, another user will die with a needle in his arm in a vacant building on Center Street off Albany Avenue, another victim of Tango and Cash. At least twenty-four other people will overdose on the new product in Hartford's north end and are taken either to Mount Sinai Hospital or Saint Francis Hospital. The deaths are not limited to Hartford, however. Five people die in New York and five in New Jersey, all attributed to the same batch of "poisonous heroin."[2] Lab testing reveals that the active ingredient isn't heroin but a much deadlier opioid: fentanyl.[3]

Fentanyl is a synthetic opioid first synthesized in 1960 by Dr. Paul Janssen, who also developed Haldol for the treatment of schizophrenia and Lomotil for the treatment of diarrhea. Fentanyl, which was approved by the US Food and Drug Administration in 1968, has a rapid onset and a short duration of action. It is initially used in surgery as an anesthetic. Later it is used for palliative care in the form of a fentanyl patch specially engineered to be placed on the skin and deliver pain relief over an extended period of time. It then comes into wide use as an alternative to morphine for quick-acting pain relief.[4] In 2010, after years of carrying only morphine in our paramedic kits, we receive fentanyl, and it soon becomes our preferred analgesic because of its rapid effect. When given intravenously, fentanyl can relieve pain in one to two minutes, with a duration of thirty to sixty minutes. The drug does not come without some controversy, though. Stories of its misuse by medical professionals are commonplace. Anesthesiologists, who have ready access to fentanyl and other opioids, are at high risk for fentanyl addiction.[5] Its abuse among medical personnel is a concern, and on-the-job deaths from fentanyl overdose are not uncommon.[6] Rumors circulate of a death on the job from fentanyl overdose at a local hospital. In 2016 and again in 2018, a nurse at Clements Hospital in Texas is found dead in a bathroom after stealing and using fentanyl.[7]

The fentanyl killing people on the streets of Hartford and across the country is not, however, medical-grade fentanyl stolen from hospital pharmacies. The fentanyl sold on the street is illegally manufactured in clandestine labs and comes mainly in the form of a white powder that is hard to distinguish visually from white powdered heroin, making it easy for dealers to add it to heroin or sell it in place of heroin. The key factor is that fentanyl is fifty to one hundred times stronger than heroin by weight (depending on the batch). In other words, 50 percent of a bag of pure heroin is likely equal in strength to 1 percent of a bag of pure fentanyl. The 12 percent pure fentanyl in Tango and Cash is roughly equivalent to twelve bags of 50 percent pure heroin. Believing they were doing the same amount of heroin they usually did, users were actually getting a dose twelve times stronger than usual. It is no wonder, then, that so many overdosed.

In 1991, finding fentanyl in street drugs is extremely rare. Investigators looking into the overdose outbreak are able to tie one batch to 126 deaths along the Eastern Seaboard. Two years after the outbreak, agents capture the person responsible for manufacturing the fentanyl in a makeshift laboratory in Wichita, Kansas. The man, George V. Marquardt, is a real-life Walter White, the antihero of the cable TV series *Breaking Bad*. A high school dropout, who once won the Wisconsin State Science Fair, Marquardt had been making drugs in his own laboratory for years. When captured, he readily admits to investigators his role in the fentanyl overdose deaths, including how he built his own spectrometer to purify his compounds. A year later, in an interview with Fusion TV, he says, "I am not a pharmacist. I am not an M.D. I'm a fellow that will manufacture a chemical compound if you have a sufficiently large quantity of money."[8]

Drug Enforcement Administration (DEA) agent Robert C. Bonner declares, "This is the only known organization manufacturing fentanyl in the United States. . . . These deadly laboratories are shut down and out-of-business."[9] For well over a decade, that is largely the case, but eventually fentanyl chemists are back to work, and this time they are working on a scale unlike any seen before.

The Centers for Disease Control and Prevention describe three waves of the current opioid epidemic.[10] The first begins in the 1990s when doctors start overprescribing pain meds. People with an injury or painful medical condition are prescribed addictive drugs in escalating doses as their tolerance increases. When they are cut off from or forced to taper the drugs, they turn to the black market to relieve the withdrawal sickness they feel. The black market is flooded with pills cranked out by the pharmaceutical companies. To increase the potency, users start crushing the pills into a powder and snorting or injecting it. The next wave begins in 2010 when Purdue Pharma comes out with tamperproof OxyContin. Users can no longer easily pulverize the pills to snort or inject. The new formula turns crushed pills into a goopy substance that is too difficult for most to contend with. It is much easier and cheaper for users to buy heroin instead. Heroin overdose deaths increase fourfold in the next five years. The third and deadliest wave begins in 2013 with the increasing adulteration of the heroin supply with illegally produced fentanyl. In 2012 fentanyl is present in only fourteen overdose deaths in Connecticut; by 2016 it is present in 479 deaths; and in 2017, for the first time, the 760 deaths attributed to fentanyl outstrip Connecticut's heroin deaths.

According to the DEA, most of the street fentanyl in the United States now comes from labs in Mexico or China. Fentanyl is smuggled into the country in the same manner that heroin is or is simply mailed to people's homes through the postal service. The fentanyl that comes directly from China is usually of high purity and is mailed in small amounts, either directly from China or via Canada. The Mexican fentanyl tends to be of lower purity. In many cases, Mexican gangs receive high-purity fentanyl from China, or make it in their own labs using chemicals from China, and then they add cut and smuggle it into the United States.[11]

There are many benefits to fentanyl from the drug dealer side of the equation. Heroin is produced from opium poppies. To produce heroin requires poppy fields that have to be cultivated. The product then has to be carried through the hills and smuggled across borders. Fentanyl's production is not affected by weather conditions, pestilence, or *federales* (Mexican federal police) destroying poppy fields. The production costs for producing a kilogram of heroin and a kilogram of fentanyl are similar. According to DEA spokesman Russ Baer, the cost of production is approximately $3,000 to $4,000 a kilo. A kilo of heroin will sell for $60,000. And fentanyl, because it is fifty times stronger than heroin, is easier to smuggle and brings in higher profits. The DEA estimates that 1 kilo of fentanyl can produce up to 24 kilos of product. That's $1.3 million in profit after it's sold to street users. The simple economics of the profit margin is what's driving the fentanyl epidemic.[12]

Today, want-to-be drug dealers without any gang affiliation can sit at home in their pajamas, drink coffee, and order fentanyl on the dark net, the part of the internet that is untraceable and requires special but publicly available software to access. They can have the drugs delivered right to their door. This allows for easy entry into the drug-dealing trade for many who otherwise would have to travel to a bad neighborhood, walk into a dimly light bar, be led to the basement, knock on a heavy door, and be checked out through the peephole. They would have to wait nervous minutes until the door finally unlatches. They would be frisked by steroid giants in muscle shirts for weapons and wires and then led into another room where the drug kingpin and his bodyguards decide whether to trust them with some of their product or just kill them instead. Meeting a guy who knows a guy who knows the man is a thing of the past.

At fifty times the strength of heroin, fentanyl is thus fifty times smaller when it comes to smuggling the same potency. Once it reaches its destination, it can then be expanded by cutting it. A bag of fentanyl sold on the street is not fifty times as strong as a bag of heroin sold on the street. The cut is different. A 50 percent pure bag of heroin (half heroin and half adulterants, or cut) equals the potency of a 1 percent pure bag of fentanyl (1 percent fentanyl and 99 percent cut). If a dealer wants to sell a bag three times as strong as a typical bag of 50 percent pure heroin, the mix has to be 3 percent fentanyl and 97 percent cut. The difficulty with fentanyl is that it has a tendency to clump, so it is much harder for a dealer to get an even mix. Like chocolate chips in cookie dough, one cookie may have more chips in it than another. One $4 bag that weighs 0.1 gram might contain 0.5 percent fentanyl, while another could contain the 12 percent strength that led to the Tango and Cash rash of overdose deaths. For many, 12 percent fentanyl is a lethal dose.

Potency also depends on the purity of the fentanyl that dealers mix with the heroin or other cut. If they have 100 percent pure fentanyl sent directly from China, they would be looking to cut it to a 1 percent purity to make it equivalent to a 50 percent bag of pure heroin. But getting it distributed evenly is not easy. Or perhaps, instead of getting 100 percent pure fentanyl, they get a batch of Mexican fentanyl that comes already cut. Maybe the powder is only 10 percent pure, so they cut it at a ratio of one to ten or less. Or maybe they don't know the purity. The point is that there is no quality control. Using any type of fentanyl is a form of Russian roulette. A fentanyl test strip will tell you that fentanyl is present, but it won't tell you how much or how pure it is.

One day Kelly tells me that when she buys bags that she knows contain fentanyl, she and her boyfriend can get gloriously high off one bag, but sometimes they buy two bags of the same product and have different reactions because the product was not well mixed. They buy Rolex, say, from the same dealer four times in a day, and each time they may get a different concentration. This variation frustrates them because they may have spent four hours raising four dollars only to get a bag that is all cut and no fentanyl. On another occasion, they may get a bag with 5 to 10 percent fentanyl, and they are quite happy. It is like hitting the lottery. Unfortunately, for some, the lottery is a death ticket.

In the past, when a bad batch of heroin hit the street, you could get a warning out: beware of Black Jack; it likely contains fentanyl. Unlike the past, though, the danger today is that, because nearly every batch has fentanyl in it and because fentanyl mixes poorly, you can have a batch with a lower than normal ratio of fentanyl overall yet still have bad bags within the batch. With fentanyl, every batch has the potential to have bad bags that will kill users if they are using alone with no one around to summon help or administer naloxone. For those who use alone, it truly is Russian roulette. A random bag may contain a deadly dose as sure as a revolver chamber may contain a fatal bullet. Because of its deadly design, fentanyl causes death rates to rise even when the number of users remains the same or declines.

I warn Kelly that the brand with a middle finger pictured on the bag has been linked to a fatal overdose. She is concerned but says she had some of that brand the day before and found it disappointing. I have this experience again with other users. While some who have tried the bags agree they are potent, others are left unsatisfied. They may not be so lucky the next time, however, if they catch a bag that should be stamped "Lethal Dose."

In Hartford, many users rely on the brand system, which flourishes in areas where many competing drug dealers need a way to distinguish their product. Some users rely on it to avoid batches they know contain fentanyl. If they prefer brown heroin, which they believe is safer, they will buy Big Doodle instead of Rolex. Some users prefer heroin for its full-bodied, organic, warm feeling as opposed to the immediate powerful rush of fentanyl. Users claim they can distinguish between heroin and fentanyl based on sight, taste (fentanyl has none), the color the drug turns when they dilute and draw it into a syringe (heroin is a darker brown), the way it makes them feel (fentanyl has a potent rush; heroin makes them itch), and duration (fentanyl doesn't last as long as heroin). Fentanyl users need another fix sooner and so end up having to buy more. Kelly prefers a mix of heroin and fentanyl; this gives her the fentanyl rush and the longer-lasting warmth of heroin. She reports, though, that such double pleasures are increasingly rare, as more and more of the bags contain only fentanyl. Her boyfriend Tom laments that there's no good heroin in Hartford anymore.

While some users avoid the dangerous fentanyl mixture, others seek it. The longer they use, the less dopamine (neurotransmitter fireworks) is produced and the lower their high becomes. They hear of a potent batch, and many feel they can handle it. To them, a batch containing fentanyl doesn't pose the risk of death but promises that long-sought-after high reminiscent of the first time they used.

Dealers play into users' mindset by having branding that suggests strength. The names stamped on bags sometimes promise to take the user beyond the brink to death itself. I find a heroin bag labeled "Dead Man"; another bag has a picture of the grim reaper on it and the words "Strike Dead." Some bags have only a skull and crossbones on them. This does not necessarily mean that these brands are the baddest of the bad. It is just marketing. Users who trust their regular dealer will probably learn what brand fits their needs.

Unfortunately, sometimes dealers have no idea what is in the mix they receive from suppliers higher up the chain. Dealers often give free samples of new product to regular users to test so that they know how much they can boast about it. This is a dangerous practice, as the users become guinea pigs. Some avoid the untested product, but others, short on cash, have no choice. Tom tells me one sample he is given makes him so dizzy and his heart race so fast that all he can do is lie down in the bushes for hours and wait for it to pass. He offers to get me a sample so I can get it tested, but I decline. I can't be carrying heroin on my person, and I am unaware of any place other than the state lab that tests samples for law enforcement cases. I do think it would be a great idea if users had a place they could take their product for testing. They could learn who is selling the good stuff and who is selling poison. That might keep the dealers honest—quality control through the street version of a better business bureau.

I hear the story of a dealer who gives out a sample of his new batch. He later calls the user to find out how he liked the product. The phone is answered by the user's mother. She hands the phone to the police officer who has responded to her home. The young man lies on the floor under a white sheet, placed on him by the paramedics who were unable to resuscitate him. Had he known his heroin was 12 percent fentanyl, he might have used more caution.

In 2016, Connecticut is one of only three states (West Virginia and Ohio are the other two) to place in the top ten nationwide for both heroin (fourth) and fentanyl (ninth) deaths per one hundred thousand people. Five of the top ten states in fentanyl deaths are in New England, with New Hampshire leading the way.[13] In 2017, for the first time, fentanyl is responsible for more deaths in Connecticut than heroin. That same year in Hartford, where Mark Jenkins is testing bags using his strips, he finds that 90 percent of the bags contain fentanyl.[14] By 2019, when the Connecticut accidental drug death toll reaches 1,200 for the year, 974 (82 percent) of the deaths involve fentanyl, while only 391 (32 percent) involve heroin. (Twenty-eight percent involve heroin and fentanyl; 53 percent involve fentanyl without heroin; and only 4 percent involve heroin with no fentanyl.)[15]

The danger of fentanyl makes harm reduction efforts even more important. A bad batch can mean death for the unsuspecting. One Friday evening, three people overdose on Green Street, one fatally. The *Hartford Courant* runs pictures of the bags police found on the scene.[16] I recognize one bag as Skull and Bones, a brand I have seen for months, mainly in the north end in roughly the same neighborhoods as the overdoses. The other bag has a design I don't recognize: two *R*s with the first one reversed. Tom Palomba, a new paramedic whom Jerry and I are training, tells us that it represents a brand of Australian blue jeans popular with youth. My suspicion is that this brand is the culprit. Kelly tells me that dealers often sell a more potent batch when introducing a new brand and then gradually weaken it with more cut once users start flocking to it. When the brand loses steam, they just put out a new and more potent brand, and the cycle continues.

A twenty-four-year-old man from one of Hartford's suburbs has his life saved by the newspaper story. The young man got into heroin five years ago through, in his own words, "stupidity." While many get into it through a doctor's prescription exposing them to opiates, he got into heroin through partying. He comes down to Hartford and buys on the street. He has a two-bundle-a-day habit (amounting to twenty bags). He doesn't inject; he snorts. He just walks down Park Street, and the dealers know what he's looking for. Pale guy with tattoos, wearing a hoodie. *We know you're not here to sample the empanadas at Aqui Me Quedo. KD? KO? Fastrack? Night Owl? High Power? We got what you're looking for.*

He gets caught up in a drug sweep once but hasn't bought his drugs yet, so after being frisked, he's let go. He nearly overdoses one time. He is on the nod on a park bench. The ambulance comes, and the paramedic gives him a good shake. He wakes up and refuses transport. He's been to rehab once and has been on Suboxone once too. He doesn't like it. A couple of weeks ago, he comes into the city, buys his heroin, and drives home. His parents don't know he is still using. His friends don't know either. There is no Narcan in his house.

Before he goes into his room to use, he picks up the newspaper his father had left on the kitchen table and brings it into the bathroom. There is the story about the triple overdose, including the fatality. He sees the pictures of the bags found at the scene. Skull and crossbones on one bag and some fancy black design with two *R*s on the other bag. The stamp catches his attention. It is the exact same design as on one of the bundles he just bought in Hartford.

You or I might immediately find Jesus, take it as a sign from above, and flush the white powder down the toilet, but he is a heroin user and needs his fix to fight off the sickness. He does what he does whenever he hears of a dangerous batch. He just does a little sample. He doesn't do the whole bundle. Maybe the guy who died hit a hot spot or had lost his tolerance. He doesn't want to overdose, so he is careful about it. You have to be. With the warning fresh in his mind, he just snorts half a bag at first. Man, it is STRONG! He finishes two bags, and he is out cold. But at least he is still breathing.

There is no knock on his bedroom door in the morning: "Son, are you okay?" No breaking the door down when his dad finds it locked and hears no answer after shouting. No hand on his cold neck feeling for an absent pulse. No call to 911. No parent doing CPR on his child. When the young man comes around in the morning, he is still in his room. No pearly gates, no fires of hell. He is still alive, and, hey, he's still got some heroin to get his day started.

That was a couple weeks ago. Today, he's sick again. He hasn't used in three days and wants help detoxing. He knows that if he doesn't get help, he will use heroin again; and one of these days, he's going to meet the batch that will kill him. We put him in the ambulance and take him from the health clinic to the hospital, and it is on the ride there that he tells me his story: "I'm looking at the paper, and I recognize the bag. I just bought that brand. I think I got to be careful. I don't want to OD. If I didn't moderate, I would have died."

Not everyone is as lucky. My partner and I are in a well-ordered apartment that clearly displays a woman's touch, with plants, neatly framed pictures, a cleanly swept floor, and a bed properly made. She spoke to her boyfriend at noon, and he was doing okay. When she got off work at five, she came home to find him in the bathroom, fully dressed, slumped on his knees, leaning over the tub, cold, blue, and stiff. They have been together for twenty years. "I got him clean," she tells me. "He's got a job. He's a good man.

Every once in a while he relapses one, two times. He just does a little 'cause he's feeling blue or his buddies give it to him. I get him straight. We got a good thing. He must have got that fentanyl shit that's killing people. I come home from work, and he's there dead. My Juan is dead."

All it takes is a lowered tolerance, a bag with a hot spot of fentanyl, and a man using alone. Just a little taste to feel better, inhale a few grains of white powder, and fifty years comes to an end on a clean bathroom floor.

Another danger of fentanyl is a syndrome known as chest wall rigidity, a rare side effect of intravenous fentanyl observed in the clinical setting. It is most likely caused by giving large amounts of fentanyl too fast, but it has also been produced by small amounts. The mechanism is not fully understood. The skeletal muscle of the chest wall stiffens, and the stiffness can extend into the abdomen, extremities, and face. Patients suffering from the syndrome are difficult to ventilate. It has been speculated that the rigidity may extend into the glottis (an area of the throat that includes the vocal cords), causing airway obstruction and a quick death. Fortunately, the syndrome responds to naloxone.

When I first heard the speculation that illicit drug users might be suffering from chest wall syndrome, I pooh-poohed it.[17] Even though I have seen the stiffening, it seemed like a hypoxic seizure as the brain is deprived of oxygen, except that it doesn't look like the hypoxic seizures I have seen in patients who seized and then went into cardiac arrest. This seizure is totally tonic—rigid muscles with no spasming—and it persists.

Most of the literature on chest wall rigidity is old, but there is a 2013 *Clinical Toxicology* article that asks the very question I am seeking to answer. The authors examined forty-eight fentanyl deaths and found that the metabolites suggested that at least half of the deaths had been rapid, consistent either with chest wall rigidity or perhaps simply a high enough dose to cause sudden respiratory arrest, followed quickly by death. They cite two pre-hospital run forms documenting difficulty with ventilating the patient until naloxone was given. It is not a very convincing article; it is mainly just speculation. But reading some of the sources the authors cite is informative.[18] One is a 1993 study published in *Anesthesiology* in which 50 percent of the human volunteers who received fentanyl at a dose of 15 micrograms per kilogram of their body weight, administered at 150 micrograms per minute, were observed to develop chest wall rigidity.[19] This dose is fifteen times the starting dose for a 220-pound patient and five times the maximum amount we would ever give one of our patients for a total dose.

Fentanyl-induced chest wall rigidity is rare in the hospital setting, but it should not be surprising to find it is a factor in overdose outside the hospital given the large amounts of fentanyl being injected. A typical $4 bag of properly mixed fentanyl sold on the streets of Hartford can be equivalent to ten 100 mcg fentanyl vials. A bag with a hot spot of fentanyl would obviously have considerably more. Some users inject up to ten bags at a time. A ten-bag dose would be one hundred times the normal hospital dose for a 220-pound man. With the poor quality control from batch to batch and even from bag to bag, I have no doubt that some users are suffering from the side effect of chest wall rigidity.

My partner and I pick up a man who appears to be on the nod, but he is breathing fine. He becomes combative when we try to get him into the ambulance. I am thinking he is high on a speedball—cocaine and heroin together. Once I close the ambulance doors, he chills out and drops off to sleep. Then I watch on the cardiac monitor as his heart rate starts to rocket, from 120 to 180 in a matter of fifteen seconds. I notice then that he has become extremely stiff like he is having a seizure, but there is no tonic-clonic activity. He has also stopped breathing. For a moment I am not certain what to do. Is it a seizure? Is this a cocaine overdose? Does he need Versed, a benzodiazepine we carry for seizures and agitation? I decide to give him a little naloxone trial: 0.4 milligrams slowly by IV. In thirty seconds, he unstiffens and is back to breathing on his own, and two minutes later he is talking to me and apologizes for causing trouble. He admits that he snorted two bags of fentanyl. At the hospital he tests positive for both fentanyl and cocaine.

A week later we respond to a call for a person who has dropped to the sidewalk right outside a treatment center. He gets immediate bystander CPR. The fire department arrives quickly, and we are there within five minutes. While I can't feel a pulse, the patient's pupils are pinpoint, and he has an irregular heartbeat rhythm on the monitor. I give him naloxone and replace the one-man bagging he was getting with the two-person method, where one person holds the mask over the face and tilts the airway so that it's properly open while the other person squeezes the bag. Within a minute, the man is breathing on his own. His carbon dioxide quickly goes down from nearly 100 to a normal 35, and his oxygen saturation goes up to 100 percent from 64. I don't give him any more naloxone, as he is breathing fine and there is no need to put him into withdrawal. I expect he will make a full recovery but am saddened to find that, despite the relatively short downtime, he has suffered a brain injury from anoxia (absence of oxygen). After a week of being made comfortable at the hospital, he passes. My suspicion is that the fentanyl caused his glottis to close, so he did not benefit from either the passive CPR ventilation he received from the bystander or the early bagging he got from the fire department.

I read a new article published in the *Harm Reduction Journal*. During a seven-month study period, staff at Insite, Vancouver's supervised injection site, responded to 1,581 overdoses and documented 497 of these people as having abnormal reactions, including 240 with muscle rigidity. The authors write, "Muscle rigidity ranged from jaw clenching to decorticate posturing with arms bent in towards the body, legs held out straight, clenched fists, and overall stiffness." In the article, they correlate the rise in abnormal reactions with the rise of fentanyl in the local drug supply. They conclude that "it is important to recognize that muscle rigidity, dyskinesia, slow or irregular heart rates, confusion, and anisocoria [pupils unequal in size] may be observed as part of overdose presentations and should still be treated with naloxone and oxygen."[20]

Fentanyl has hit New England, the Midwest, and Appalachia hard, but it has yet to become a huge factor in most of the United States west of the Mississippi. Fentanyl is easy to mix in or sell in place of powdered heroin, which is commonplace in the East. In the West, much of the heroin available is black-tar heroin, a hard or sticky tarlike substance that is crudely processed from the opium poppy. It is either smoked or injected after being diluted and heated. It is harder to adulterate with fentanyl; however, should powdered heroin move west in significant quantities or dealers find better ways to add fentanyl to black-tar heroin during processing, expect death rates in western states to skyrocket as they have in the East. The economics that drives suppliers to use fentanyl instead of heroin should eventually apply nationwide in the United States. A 2019 report by the RAND Corporation warns that, nationally, the synthetic opioid problem "is likely to get worse before it gets any better."[21]

It hasn't come to Hartford yet in a measurable way, but emergency responders in states such as Michigan, West Virginia, Florida, and particularly Ohio[22] have encountered patients who have overdosed on heroin laced with carfentanil, an opioid of the synthetic fentanyl family that is ten thousand times stronger than morphine (one hundred times stronger than fentanyl) and usually used to tranquilize elephants, grizzly bears, and large elk. It is also suspected that the Russian army uses it as a chemical weapon.

In October of 2002, a group of armed Chechens take eight hundred hostages who are attending a musical at a local Russian theater. The rebels demand an end to the Chechen war and the withdrawal of all Russian troops from their country or else they will execute all the hostages. On the fourth day of the siege, Russian troops pump an unknown chemical into the theater's ventilation ducts. The gas quickly renders people unconscious and kills 129 of the hostages and 39 of the attackers by stopping their respiration. Experts will later decide that the gas was likely carfentanil.[23] Had the Russians had a sufficient supply of naloxone on hand, they could have saved most of the victims. Because they did not, many died.

On YouTube there is a recording of a phone conversation between an older man inside a Florida jailhouse, Robert Rigby, and his twenty-five-year-old girlfriend, Melissa Winings.[24] Rigby tells her in code how to mix the drugs they have at home to avoid causing overdoses in any more of their customers. The key ingredient is potent, so she needs to be extremely careful. "Will you do that for me from now on, not guesstimate and use those numbers?" he asks her. "Yes, baby," she answers. She either doesn't or can't follow instructions, and the first customer she sells the new mix to falls over dead immediately after using. The medical examiner confirms that the user died from carfentanil.[25]

The problem with carfentanil is that it's so potent. One hundred times stronger than fentanyl, a bag of carfentanil needs to be only 0.01 percent pure to be the equivalent in strength to a 50 percent pure bag of heroin or a 1 percent pure bag of fentanyl. The difficulty in mixing carfentanil and the enormous danger in getting it wrong may be enough of a deterrent to keep carfentanil from ever displacing fentanyl as the chief killer of the opioid epidemic.

If, however, underground chemists can find a way to dilute carfentanil in liquid in a manner that ensures reasonable survival rates, the overdose situation may change again for the worse.

Adding chemical-weapon-grade powder to product is a horrifying development in the opioid epidemic. But when I think about it more, I don't know that I'm inclined to reserve a special place in hell for dealers who do it. Where they are going, they will have company. How different are their practices from those of mainstream businesses that ignore or hide evidence of their products causing cancer, heart disease, or obesity, or even having the capacity of maiming or killing? No difference, in my opinion. And you can't accuse the heroin dealers of false advertising, particularly when they brand their product with names and imagery of danger and death: Strike Dead, R.I.P., Dead Man, Black Widow, Pray for Death, Skull and Bones.

Contrast drug dealers' marketing with Purdue Pharma's advertising for OxyContin. In an ad series called I Got My Life Back, the company interviewed employed people who were smiling and boasting of how great they feel. Sadly, in a follow-up documentary, the wife of one of the I Got My Life Back participants tells how her husband's life deteriorated. He seemed overmedicated all the time, and he eventually fell asleep at the wheel of his car and died in a crash.[26] If drug dealers made videos, they might show their customers being tossed into graves with warning signs flashing on the screen. No deception there.

Let me ask you, Who is more accountable? The kid from a broken home who went to an overcrowded school, dropped out, and makes money the only way he knows how, by slinging $4 bags of heroin to people who seek him out? Or the CEO of a pharmaceutical company who grew up with every advantage, went to an Ivy League school, got a job from a family friend making six figures to start, earns multimillions plus stock options, knows his product is addicting and killing hundreds of thousands, but hides that fact as he keeps on pushing it? Why should one go away for twenty years and the other only have to pay a fine that won't even affect his country-club lifestyle?

Some heroin dealers in Hartford have switched up their drug stamps to celebrate Halloween. Drug users are being treated to brands such as Killer Clowns, Freddy vs. Jason, and Casper (the Friendly Ghost). Here are questions for the users on Halloween: Does their $4 wax envelope contain a trick or a treat? Are they getting heroin or fentanyl? And what has it been cut with: brown sugar, baby formula, Benadryl, rat poison, caffeine, paracetamol, chloroquine, quinine, flour, chalk, talcum powder, sucrose, starch, powdered milk, acetaminophen, or carfentanil? Will the bag get them high, or will it kill them?

I wonder, as well, if the dealers wear a *Scream* mask on Halloween. Do they dress like a killer clown? Do they wear a Donald Trump mask, or are they dressed like Superman? Do they hang paper skeletons and carve and light a jack-o'-lantern to guide users to their drug lair? I also wonder about the Big Pharma executives. What do they do on Halloween night? Do they also wear a *Scream* mask when little children come to their door? Would they even think of putting razor blades in the apples they give out? Stone pebbles in boxes of candy corns? Or rat poison in place of sugar powder in Pixy Stix? Certainly not, but then why do they not provide fair warning to the public of the dangers of the product that paid for their mansion?

Responder Safety

Fentanyl can be deadly to users when injected into a vein, inhaled and absorbed through the nasal mucosa, or ingested in sufficient quantities. But what are the dangers to first responders who may come into incidental contact with the powder?

In EMS, responders are taught *scene safety*. Responders don't go running into a scene just because someone has called for help. If a woman calls, screaming that she is being beaten up by her boyfriend, EMTs wait at the curb until the police secure the scene. If a house is on fire, EMTs do not run inside unless they are also firefighters who have the proper protective response gear. You have to be alive to save someone else. This is drilled into you in EMS class. When you are tested with mock scenarios such as cardiac arrest or multisystem trauma, you must first state, "Scene safety—BSI," which stands for body substance isolation, or else you automatically fail the station no matter how well you know your medicine and paramedic skills. You have to protect yourself first.

In June 2016, the federal Drug Enforcement Administration (DEA) releases a two-minute video, *Fentanyl: A Real Threat to Law Enforcement.*[1] Jack Riley, the deputy administrator, opens the video by stating that "a very small amount [of fentanyl] ingested or absorbed through your skin can kill you." He introduces two police detectives who describe their experience with a fentanyl exposure. One detective describes how, in sealing a baggie of the drug, some of it "poofed up" into the air, and the detectives ended up inhaling it. "I felt like my body was shutting down," the other detective says. "People around me say I looked really white and lost color. And it just really felt like . . . I thought that was it. I thought I was dying. That's what my body felt like. If I could imagine or describe a feeling where your body is completely shutting down, and, you know, preparing to stop, stop living, you know, that's the feeling I felt." The first detective adds, "You actually felt like you were dying. You couldn't breathe, very disoriented. Everything you did was exaggerated in your mind, I guess. It was the most bizarre feeling that I never ever would want to feel again. And it was just a little bit of powder that just puffed up in the air." Riley concludes, "Fentanyl can kill you."

As I watch it, I think about being a paramedic for more than twenty-five years. What they are describing doesn't sound like an opioid overdose. People who use heroin describe it as the most wonderful feeling they have ever experienced. They feel euphoria. The comedian Lenny Bruce described it as like kissing God. They give up everything they have to "chase the dragon." What these detectives are describing doesn't sound like an opioid reaction; it sounds like anxiety.

A year later the DEA updates its video. This time Chuck Rosenberg, the acting administrator of the DEA, proclaims, "Fentanyl is deadly. Exposure to an amount equivalent to even a few grains of sand can kill you. You can be in grave danger if you unintentionally come into contact with fentanyl. It can be absorbed into the bloodstream through your skin."

The DEA also releases *Fentanyl: A Briefing Guide for First Responders*. It includes the following passage:

Personnel should look for any cyanosis (turning blue or bluish color) of victims, including the skin or lips, as this could be a sign of fentanyl overdose caused by respiratory arrest. Further, before proceeding, personnel should examine the scene for any loose powders (no matter how small), as well as nasal spray bottles, as these could be signs of fentanyl use.

Opened mail and shipping materials located at the scene of an overdose with a return address from China could also indicate the presence of fentanyl, as China-based organizations may utilize conventional and/or commercial means to ship fentanyl and fentanyl-related substances to the United States.[2]

I have to read the passage several times to make certain I understand it. I focus on one key phrase: "Before proceeding." The DEA is saying that before treating a person with agonal respirations—someone moments from dying—emergency personnel should check the scene for packages from China.

I write on my EMS blog, "If a patient is unresponsive and cyanotic, breathing two times a minute, unless they have fallen into a Scarface mountain of powder or any amount of powder that I think might compromise my ability to perform my duty of saving their life, I am going to put my gloves on, don my N-95 mask, grab my bag-valve-mask and start breathing for them. I am most certainly not going to wait to treat the patient until after I have scoured the cluttered room for hidden packages from China."[3]

Scene safety is important, yes, but unless you are in a legitimate hazmat scene, it is misguided to let a person die while you look for possible powder that, if left undisturbed, will not harm anyone. If, on the other hand, everyone on the scene is either unmoving on the floor or the powder is so thick on the ground that you can leave footprints in it, then I am going to turn around and exit.

On July 26, 2017, the *Los Angeles Times*, in a story about a drug overdose scene, warns that "a small dose of the odorless white powder can be fatal." The story describes the police response to an overdose call: "Officers have been trained to 'back off' when they come across white powder and an unconscious victim at the scene of a call."[4] It is unclear from the article how long treatment was delayed to the three overdose victims, one of whom died. My hope is that medics, with proper personal protective equipment (PPE), were allowed to go right in to treat the patients. Police corporal Bertagna is quoted as saying, "A woman and three children were also found in the 800-square-foot apartment and removed." Bertagna continues: "They, along with the officers and paramedics, all underwent decontamination, essentially an intense shower." The fact that a woman and three children were alert in the same apartment suggests that the scene was likely safe.

The next day, the *Wall Street Journal* runs this front-page article: "Fentanyl Isn't Just Deadly for Drug Users: Police Are Getting Sickened."[5] The article is fascinating for its details on how fear of the drug has transformed the way that everyone, from local cops to medical examiners to prosecutors, handle their business. The article cites the cases of an Ohio officer who collapsed after brushing powder off his shirt and a Maryland officer who had naloxone sprayed into his nose while he was still conscious and talking. The Ohio case generates an article in *Slate* magazine written by a toxicologist titled "The Viral Story about the Cop Who Overdosed by Touching Fentanyl Is Nonsense."[6] In the Maryland case, the officer felt his heart racing after seeing a white substance and had fellow responders squirt him with naloxone while he was still talking. The article mentions how the responders never bothered to attach the atomizer to the syringe of naloxone because they were so panicked that there wasn't time enough to save him.[7] Needless to say, this officer does not meet the guidelines for administering naloxone, and getting naloxone as a liquid, without it being atomized into a mist, severely limits its effectiveness, unless it is being used as a placebo.

When all we have are newspaper accounts, which can be inaccurate, the most we can do is comment on the facts reported. There is clearly an atmosphere of fear in these articles. The danger of spreading bad information is that critical care will be delayed because of unwarranted fear. The specter of a pile of fentanyl powder suddenly morphing into a devilish cloud that strikes down a brigade of responders is science fiction. Leave the powder be, wear PPE, and take care of the human being in respiratory depression.

What is the logical extension of the DEA's reasoning? There are millions of users in the country who inhale or inject powdered heroin and fentanyl multiple times a day. Are they all walking hazmat scenes? Could they have grains of powder in their clothing? Does this mean that a patient with a history of heroin use should be treated like an Ebola patient, requiring an isolation room, decontamination, and health personnel donning and doffing high-level protective gear, all because of the misguided belief that touching the powder can kill?

I correspond with a law enforcement agent who is curious to know whether I am seeing a bag marked "KD" on the street. KD, which stands for basketball player Kevin Durant, is the brand behind a fatality that resulted in a man going to prison. Yes, I tell her, the brand is still out there. When I run into her at a conference, I ask if she has ever seen the bag up close. I have an empty KD wrapper in my wallet to give her as a souvenir. I move to pull it out of my wallet, and she puts her hands up. Given her reaction, I stop what I am doing. I don't want the conference hotel lobby to turn into the scene from *ET* where the house is cordoned off and men barge in wearing hazmat suits.

On July 30, an article in the *Eagle-Tribune* of North Andover, Massachusetts, describes a town spending $75,000 on a hazmat response to a scene where three people overdosed. The article includes this line: "The fear on Garden Street that morning was the men had overdosed on either fentanyl or carfentanil, an even stronger man-made opioid that can be toxic to someone merely in its presence."[8] There is no scientific evidence that fentanyl or carfentanil is toxic to anyone who is merely in the same room as the drug. The danger is inhalation or injection. If you wear PPE, there is little risk in treating your patients.

On July 27, 2017, the American College of Medical Toxicology and the American Academy of Clinical Toxicology issue a joint statement, *Preventing Occupational Fentanyl and Fentanyl Analog Exposure to First Responders*, stating that "the risk of clinically significant exposure to emergency responders is extremely low."[9]

Many people are prescribed fentanyl patches by their doctor for pain relief. The patches are specially engineered to enter the bloodstream through the skin. They include a special preparation that allows the drug to get through the skin, but it takes hours to do so and requires large doses. Mere grains of powder will not enter the body simply by coming into contact with the skin. A toxicologist tells me that you would have to sit in a bathtub of powder for a long time for it to work its way through your skin.

Jonathan Swift, the satirist and author of *Gulliver's Travels* wrote, "Falsehood flies, and truth comes limping after it, so that when men come to be undeceived, it is too late; the jest is over, and the tale hath had its effect." Dr. Charles McKay, a respected toxicologist, shared this quotation with me. He had thought of it after reading some news accounts of the public safety response to possible fentanyl overdose scenes. The falsehood that just touching fentanyl can kill you has persisted despite the joint statement from the toxicology associations.

When giving a presentation at a conference, I suggest that if fentanyl is as dangerous on contact as it's claimed to be, we will need to put yellow tape around the city of Hartford because of the prevalence of heroin bags on the ground. I play a game with my partners: no matter where we take the ambulance on a call in the city, I can always find a heroin wrapper within fifty feet of the vehicle. On Park Street we shrink it to ten feet.

In September 2017, the acting head of the DEA, Chuck Rosenberg, when speaking at a Yale Law School opioid conference, repeats the DEA's party line on fentanyl. "It will kill you," he says. And for those with no tolerance, Rosenberg warns, "It can kill you to the touch."[10]

In the November 2017 issue of the *American Journal of Emergency Medicine*, in an article about the controversies surrounding carfentanil, fentanyl, and other fentanyl analogs, the physician authors take the DEA and the media to task for sensationalizing the dangers that these synthetic opioids pose to responders. They write that the DEA's claim that mucosal or dermal absorption of fentanyl can kill rapidly, and the DEA's video of two officers describing their symptoms following accidental exposure, should "be treated with healthy skepticism." They note that the officers' symptoms are "inconsistent with opioid poisoning." They also note that "it is unquestionable that both drug users and sellers contact the product on a regular basis without apparent harm."[11]

Misinformation and inconsistent recommendations for fentanyl continue to result in confusion among first responders. It seems that every week responders are getting exposed to fentanyl, being rushed to the hospital, with many getting Narcan, all often without exhibiting any symptoms or symptoms no worse than light-headedness and tingling hands. One headline reads, "Officers Hospitalized after Becoming Dizzy and Feeling 'A Tingling Sensation' at the Scene of Fatal Fentanyl Overdose."[12] Another one reads, "Cops Left Dizzy and Numb after Exposure to Mysterious Substance during NC Drug Search."[13] I have been told at scenes to be careful because just touching a speck of powder could kill me. No, I say, that's not true.

Finally, in April 2018, the Office of National Drug Control Policy releases a new set of recommendations along with a video to dispel the confusion.[14] One scene in the video, called *Fentanyl: The Real Deal*, tells it all. A police officer gets some powder on his hands and screams, "I got some on my hands!" and then gets all woozy, with special effects distorting the officer's face.

His female partner shakes her head at his silliness. She tells him, "Wash your hands. You'll be okay." And he is fine.[15]

Here's the bottom line for layperson and responder alike: Touching fentanyl will not kill you. If you get it on your hands, don't touch your nose or eyes. Wash your hands with soap. Wear gloves. If there is powder in the air, wear a mask and eye protection. You do not need to get Narcan sprayed up your nose just because you were exposed. Only give naloxone to someone who is breathing too slowly (hypoventilating) and who has true signs of opioid toxidrome (such as pinpoint pupils and depressed mental status). People who are awake and breathing rapidly (hyperventilating) do not need naloxone. EMS responders should follow their treatment protocols.

Not long after the new recommendations are released, a local drug suspect fleeing a bust attempts to throw a large bag of heroin out the window of the building, but the window is closed. The powder goes up in the air in a miasmic cloud, and a couple of officers get some on them. One of my company's ambulances on standby is besieged by panicked officers demanding Narcan, which the EMTs provide. The officers dose themselves and then head back into the building.

Falsehood flies.

Family

In the opioid crisis, families need support as they struggle to understand what is happening to their loved one. It is hard to imagine the fear they face when a loved one disappears. A son or daughter may go out to the store, yet as the hours tick off, the family fears the worst.

A young man is in his parents' Subaru parked to the side of a gas station near the highway ramps. The car is running, in drive, his foot on the brake. He is slumped forward against the wheel. This sight aroused the attention of passersby who called 911. We arrive within minutes. We try to open the doors, which are locked. Jerry bangs hard on the driver side window, while I go to the passenger side and bang on that window. I notice through the tinted window a second person in the passenger seat, also slumped over. Our banging causes the driver to stir. He opens his eyes, frightened. He moves his hand to the gearshift but then realizes he already has it in drive. He tries to go forward, but a bus is blocking the intersection. A police officer arrives and is also yelling and banging on the car: "Stop the car! Stop the car!"

He puts the car in park and freezes. People are shouting and banging on the car. He is a trapped animal. Finally, slowly, he surrenders. He unlocks the door. The police officer opens it and yanks him out of the car. The police officer has the young man put his arms behind his back. There is shouting: "Where's your sharp? Where's your sharp?"

I open the passenger door now, which unlocked when the driver's door opened. The man slumped in the passenger seat looks up slowly. His face is hardened and weathered. His pupils are pinpoint; he's drowsy. I recognize him as a user whom I've seen shuffling up and down the streets and through the parks of the city. Another police officer arrives and hails the man by name: "Hey, Charlie, what are you doing in this car? Who's your friend?"

"Bart," he says. "Bart."

"Bart? Really. You giving Bart a tour of the city, huh? You're a tour guide, showing him all the neighborhoods? Is he buying your heroin for you?"

I see the needle on the floor of the car and reach in and pick it up. I take it back to the ambulance and dispose of it in the sharps box. Both passengers are out of the car now and being frisked.

Bart is a short, skinny, pale-faced boy of nineteen from a suburb. He is wearing blue Flintstones pajama bottoms, a New York Giants t-shirt, and sneakers without socks. His hair is dirty and matted. He is crying as the officer shouts at him. He finally admits to doing two bags of heroin with Charlie. On the floor of the car are two torn bags. One is stamped "Sony"; the other is red and possibly reads "The Flash," although the stamp is faded.

Charlie is trying to persuade the officer to let him retrieve his backpack from the car because it contains all he owns in the world. He says he doesn't need to go to the hospital. Amid the chaos, Bart ends up in the back of the ambulance, his car gets hooked to a tow truck, and his passenger takes off down the street. No one is arrested.

In the ambulance, I try to console Bart. His parents are going to be so disappointed in him, he says. He was doing so well. He was on Suboxone and hadn't used in months. If only Charlie hadn't called him.

I find out how Bart knows Charlie. Bart happened to be in a car in Hartford another time, also at a gas station after having bought two bags of heroin from a contact a classmate had told him about. Charlie saw Bart snorting the drug, so he came over and suggested that Bart might want to try injecting. The high is much better, he told him. Soon the two of them were meeting. Charlie would provide the drug; Bart would pay for it; and Charlie would help Bart inject to make certain he found a vein. Today Bart paid Charlie $25 for half a bundle. A bundle is typically $30 and contains ten bags. I do the math for Bart: "So you guys did two bags? You paid him $25? Where are the other three bags?"

Bart looks confused.

"And let me ask you something else," I add. "You both injected, right?"

Bart confirms.

"But I found only one syringe," I say.

There is silence.

"Tell me you didn't," I say.

More silence.

"You two shared the needle?"

Bart nods glumly.

"Jesus Christ!" I say. "You can't do that."

"He only had one needle."

I want to say, What were you thinking? But I know not all users think. The wiring in their brain has gone screwy. They lack the ability to judge risk. "Do you have Narcan at home?" I ask.

"No."

"You need to have Narcan with you wherever you go. Your parents need to have it in your house."

"But I was in recovery. I wasn't going to do heroin anymore."

"That doesn't matter. People relapse despite having the best intentions. You need to get it, and your parents need to have it. And you need to use clean needles. Your pal Charlie in all likelihood has hepatitis C and maybe HIV. He has been around the block. Addiction is hard, but you need to protect yourself."

Bart returns to sobbing. I hand him a Kleenex and feel bad for upsetting him. At the same time, I know the young man needs serious counseling. I have no doubt that Bart's parents love him, and I know that Bart and his parents face a long road ahead. "You can't recover if you're dead," I say. "We need to get you help." I then ask Bart, as I ask all of my patients, how he got started on this path.

"I tore my ACL skateboarding three years ago," Bart says.

"Your doctor prescribed you pain meds?"

"I got hooked on them."

"You took more than you should?"

Bart nods: "They made me feel better."

The path he traveled is one that many others have trod. Buying pain meds is expensive. He was introduced to heroin, which he could snort and which was cheaper. He started coming in to Hartford. Then he met Charlie, and his habit became serious. His family put him into rehab, and when he got out, he was taking Suboxone. An opioid that lasts much longer than heroin, it moderates cravings and can help people stay away from heroin. He said he was doing really well. Just the day before, in fact, he had helped his grandfather paint his garage. Then Charlie called, and Bart slipped up. He couldn't resist the thought of getting that heroin high again. Now he is in the ambulance, and his parents' car is on the back of a tow truck. When they find out, they are going to be so disappointed in him.

Bart blubbers. He is a nineteen-year-old boy in blue Flintstones pajama bottoms, with paint still on his hands from helping his grandfather. My partner and I help get Bart into a room in the ED, find him a blanket and pillow, and wish him well. We remind him about the need to have Narcan available, to use clean needles, and to never shoot up alone.

I tell the ED nurse that Bart has no Narcan at home and that he shared a needle with a known IV drug user. I ask the ED team to reinforce the messages about Narcan and the need for clean needles. The young nurse, who is very busy, says, "That's rehab's job. And he should know better."

"If you take the time to treat him like a human being and try to help him, you may keep him from coming back to the ED and inconveniencing you."

"I'm sorry," she says. "They just gave me two other patients, and I'm swamped."

"No doubt," I say. I understand that she is under stress, and no one works as hard as ED nurses. But Bart's sickness is real, and his story is tragic. I don't want his parents to get a phone call one day telling them he is dead. He can be helped if people pay attention to him.

We are worried that Bart will simply be observed and then discharged, but in fact he is admitted to the substance abuse wing. While he is being admitted, he tries to escape. He flees the hospital shirtless, wearing just his blue pajama bottoms. But it is cold out on this November day, and he has nowhere to go. He turns around and knocks on the ED door. They take him back in.

Bart's family will get a phone call that he is at the ED, and it will likely crush them that he has relapsed, but at least he is still alive in the world. His chance of recovery one day remains a possibility.

We are in the lot at 1200 Park. Kelly has come over and is talking to us. I still stock the ambulance with oranges and protein bars so that I have something to give her and some of the other users I talk with. It is startling sometimes to see how quickly they will devour an apple or an orange, as though they haven't eaten in weeks. Gauging from the lack of body fat on many of the users, I would imagine that's often not too far from the truth.

While Kelly chows down on a chocolate protein bar, we watch Randy, a tall young man in his early twenties with sunburned skin and surfer blond hair, scream at a well-dressed woman who has just gotten out of an Oldsmobile. "That's his mom," Kelly says. "They are always fighting." Randy is a regular in the plaza. While Kelly sits quietly by the store exit and relies on people offering her change, or does small chores for them like folding their laundry in the laundromat or carrying their groceries to their car, Randy goes aggressively from car to car, begging for money. He thrusts an empty soda cup at people and seems to do well at it.

"He's got it great," Kelly says. "He stays under the highway with us and then spends his weekends at his mom's house in Wethersfield, sleeping in his own bed, getting home-cooked meals. She gives him money and even drives him to Park Street to buy his drugs." The woman turns her back on him and walks back to the car. He stalks after her, yelling. I am rooting for her to get in the car and drive away, but she doesn't. She ends up handing him some bills and hugging him. "Always the drama," Kelly says.

I wonder about Kelly's parents. She tells me they want nothing more to do with her. Her mother is a prescription drug addict; her stepfather doesn't care for her. She hasn't seen her real father in years. Her mother and stepfather told her not to come around anymore as long as Tom, her boyfriend, is with her. They think he is the cause of her problems. Kelly has three kids of her own, all scattered and living with relatives. She calls them sometimes using Skype on her phone when she has one. She uses the Wi-Fi at the laundromat. I offer to lend her my phone to FaceTime with them, but she always has an excuse not to. She tells me once that she and Tom are going to see the kids at Christmas. A relative is going to pick them up, and they are going to go out to eat together, but then the visit never happens. A few days before Christmas, I ask Tom about their Christmas plans. He is the father of Kelly's youngest child. "When's Christmas?" he responds. Kelly tells me that she knew she was relapsing and left; she didn't want her kids to see her like that. I know she loves them because her face lights up whenever she talks about them. Sometimes she talks about a future where she and Tom have a little house and jobs, she regains custody of her kids, and they all live together as a family. But her reverie is short-lived. In the moment, it seems that all she can focus on is rounding up $4 to get her next bag of heroin. I wonder if her mother ever dreams about a day when they are all back together or if she truly has given up on her.

I hope I never have to confront this addiction with one of my daughters. I don't think I would be capable of tough love. If one of my daughters was going to overdose, I would much rather have her overdose in her own bed than under a highway somewhere where no one might find her for days.

Thanksgiving is coming up, and Veronica is hoping that a friend will take her out to the countryside so she can surprise her sister. She says she is down to only two bags a day yet can't quite break free. Inez, a thin woman in her fifties who sits in front of the bakery every day hoping people will give her spare change or pay her to wash their car, wants to go see her father in Bridgeport, but she says she is ashamed for him to see her the way she is. She doesn't want to break his heart. It has been seven years since she has been home.

A woman on a cell phone stands outside a car. She explains to us that the male in the car has been smoking crack, taking benzos, and doing heroin for several days. I ask her if he's breathing. She says yes, but he is asleep right now. When she picked him up at his friend's house in their suburban town an hour earlier, he was out cold. His friends were going to give him Narcan, but the girl with them said not to waste it. The girl then punched him hard in the chest twice and put ice in his pants. I ask the woman with the cell phone what her relationship is to the person in the car. "He is my son," she says.

I approach the car. A heavily tattooed man wearing basketball shorts and an NBA jersey is fully reclined in the passenger seat. His mouth is open, and his eyes are shut. I can't tell whether he's breathing. A police officer is standing next to me now. He opens the front door. I open the back door. I consider for a moment using the line from the *Lil' Dope Fiend* comic book: "I'm going to Narcan you! I'm taking all your dope!" Instead, though, I give the young man the traditional sternal rub. He springs forward. "What? What the fuck!" he says. "What's going on?" He is in his mid-twenties, a powerfully built, thick-necked young man with short hair and missing teeth. "What the fuck, Mom? Where did you take me? Hartford? The cops? Really, Mom! Really?"

"You need help," she says. "You need rehab, and your foot is infected."

"My foot is infected. Yeah, my foot is infected. I'm a drug addict, Mom. Of course, it's infected!"

The officer says, "I've dealt with you before. What's your name?"

"Not me."

"No, I'm sure I have."

"It was probably my brother. We look alike. People mistake us."

"Maybe."

The mother says, "You need to let them take you to the hospital."

"No, I'm not going to the hospital. You're taking me back to my boys. I can't believe you did this?"

"I'm not taking you back. You either go to the hospital, or you can walk home."

"Walk home? It's twenty miles! I don't have socks. You're going to leave me here on my own in Hartford without socks and shoes!"

"You have shoes right there." I point to the sneakers by his feet.

"These aren't my shoes! Jesus, Mom, you could have at least grabbed my socks!"

"Maybe it's 'cause your feet are swollen."

"I told you I'm a drug addict."

"He injects in his feet," his mother says. "He just got treated for an infection, but it's worse."

"Please, dude," he says to the cop. "Make her take me back to my boys. That's cold what she did."

"It's between you and your mom."

"I don't want you in my car," she says. "I don't want to see you anymore. I am done with you and your brother both."

"Fine, but give me a ride back to my boys. You brought me down here; now take me back!"

"Your mom wants you out of the car," the officer says, "It's her car. You have to get out."

"But I have no socks. That's not fair."

"It's not fair," the officer says, "but you're a man, you have to deal with it."

"Mom, just take me back to my boys."

"I can't take this any longer," the mother says.

"I have no fucking socks!"

This goes on for about fifteen minutes. In between, there are some actions. He knows where he is, the date, and the president. He denies suicidal thoughts. He tries to light the butt of a cigarette found on the floorboard. His mom says he is going to kill himself. He misses all his rehab appointments. He apologizes for that, sincerely he says, but says he is still not getting out of the car. She is worried about the fentanyl and the elephant drug (carfentanil). And she can't spend her nights looking for him anymore. She is sixty years old, she says, and she is tired. With the son still refusing to get out of the car, I tell his mom how to get Narcan by going to the pharmacy and getting the pharmacist to write her a prescription on the spot. Insurance will pay for it, except for a small copay. She should always have it on her, I tell her. But she doesn't allow her sons in her house anymore, she says. But you're still involved with them, I say. Yes, she nods, she is.

He now says that he hasn't eaten for days. We again bring up the hospital and say that he can get a hot meal there and get his foot looked at.

"I'm not going to the fucking hospital. I got to get back to my boys!"

"All right, all right," the mother finally says. "I'll take you back to your boys if you just shut up. After that, I'm done with you!" The officer asks her if she is sure, if she feels safe with him. "He is my son," she says. I tell her again how to get Narcan and to keep it in her purse. She nods and says she'll do it. She gets in the car. "Put your seat belt on," she says to her son. He shakes his head but puts the seat belt on.

They drive off.

We have a small Thanksgiving celebration at my house. I cook a turkey too big for us all to eat. At the halftime of a football game, I put away the last of the food in the refrigerator. I think briefly about driving to Park Street and passing out turkey and pie to the homeless users I know. (I bring food to Kelly and Tom the next day. Later Kelly tells me to thank my daughter for the brownies, but she admits that the fat on the turkey led to stomach distress.) Instead we walk to a nearby park. My kids and I kick a soccer ball and play in the orange and yellow leaves. I think of families at wakes, standing solemnly in line as people come to pay their respects. On the table are pictures of the lost child, including one taken on a day like this. I want to hold time still.

Partners

Janis frequents the park on Hudson Street. I see her at times smoking a cigarette while she sits on one of the playground swings. Many nights she sleeps on cardboard by the fence; on rainy nights she ties one end of a tarp to the fence and weights the other end on the grass to provide shelter. She is tall and gawky with red hair and looks a lot older than her early thirty-something years because she has lost most of her teeth. Nothing makes a person look older than receded gums. I see her one morning in the summer when the temperature is already up into the eighties, and the humidity makes it hard to breathe. I ask her if she wants a water, which she does. She smiles in such a way that I can see her youth hasn't been completely driven from her body by the hard living she has put it through. I also give her an orange and a couple of bucks. She has a tattoo of a blue pony on her neck. It is faded, but the pony looks like a kid's magical pony, the kind that can fly when it isn't being cuddled by a four-year-old.

I don't know too much about her. I know her name is Janis and know she's a heroin user. But I don't know the backstory of how she lost her teeth—whether through disease, accident, or someone slugging her in the mouth. I don't know how she came to call the small park her home. She rarely goes down to Pope Park, where we sometimes post our ambulance and where I get to know many of the users walking east up Park Street to buy their drugs. I usually see her walking alone, going in and out of a bodega or standing on the corner lighting a cigarette. Even among the murals and store signs on Park Street, her hair stands out like Technicolor in the old movies. I wonder if she is close to anyone on these streets, if she has any friends, anyone to look out for her.

Having a partner not only can be lifesaving if the partners use together, but it also helps users feel like they are still part of the human fabric. The only downside, and it is a considerable one, is that it takes two willing partners or one exceptionally strong individual to commit to recovery.

I drive Park Street each day, watching the people block by block. Some pull over in their car to buy quickly from a street-side dealer. Homeless users, who I have watched beg for money, walk up the street counting their change. A stream of gaunt, sunken-eyed people with tattoos and backpacks walk into the alley behind the Bean Pot Restaurant. Later, I see them head for the park. Some go into the bushes to use; others sit on the park benches or go down to the pavilion by the pond. Some users are solo; others are always in pairs.

A tall, broad-shouldered man and a smaller thin man I see regularly. The taller man, who always wears a muscle shirt, has a New York Yankees tattoo on his shoulder. Aside from their different sizes, they look almost like brothers.

I am in the bakery one day getting a pernil (roast pork) sandwich. While the girl behind the counter puts the long flat sandwich in the presser for me, I listen to the two of them talk. "You promised me I could have a guava jelly," the younger one says.

"And I'm going to get it for you; just be patient there, Lenny," the bigger man replies. "We're going to order the coffee first like we always do. Then you can pick out whatever pastry you want." The tall hefty one, Berto, is sharper; the shorter one, Lenny, seems slow. They are never apart.

One day I see them unloading a truck in front of one of the markets. Berto is doing most of the work. I imagine the driver slips him a ten when they are done and maybe gives Lenny a five. Another day we are out on a call on Park Street. A man is standing asleep on his feet, on the serious nod. While my partner gives him a little shake, not to startle him, but enough to get him to open his eyes, I see a man walking fast down the street carrying a case of Corona beer. It strikes me as odd, as I know him to be an opioid user. Why would he be spending his money on so much beer? Then I see Lenny also carrying a case, although he is struggling with his. Then the big fellow Berto comes lumbering along, sidestepping, with three cases of Corona in his massive arms, the third case he has balanced against his face. Almost immediately, this turns into a flood of people scurrying down the sidewalk carrying cases of Corona. I look up the street and see a beer truck parked in front of the liquor store, with the driver slowly unloading cases onto his dolly. On the other side of the truck, neighborhood folk have opened up a side cargo door and are stripping him of his load. One of the firefighters who has arrived on our call catches on and starts shouting to the driver. The driver runs around to the other side, only to see the last of the bandits fleeing down the block and disappearing into the brush behind the old abandoned charity center.

I imagine Berto and Lenny telling the tale to their other street buddies and guzzling a beer or two, until they realize that what they really need to do is sell what they have left to buy their next bags of heroin. While I don't condone the theft, and feel bad for the driver, who hopefully won't have to pay for the theft out of his own paycheck, the comic nature of the crime makes me laugh, and I also liked seeing the joy on the bandits' faces. I am glad for Berto and Lenny that they have each other.

In Pope Park, a couple shooting up in their battered Ford smile and show me their Narcan as I walk by. He looks to be in his thirties, a muscular man with a beard and Boston Red Sox hat. She is maybe in her midtwenties, with long black hair and beautiful eyes. I try not to stare at her. She looks like the nurse in *ER*, who later became the star of *The Good Wife*. I look at her and think, my god, what happened? How did she get so led astray? A month later I see them walking together and carrying what's left of their belongings in backpacks and shopping bags. After buying, they walk down the hill and into the woods to where a circle of brownstone lies, on the edge of a meadow. It was an old meeting place for Hartford settlers, now a meeting place for users. Often over the next several months, I see them together there and up on Park Street, and each time I see them, they look worse, faces burned by the sun, eyes hollowed, skin stretched tight over their bones. I wonder when they first met, how they came together, and what their trajectories will be. Then I see only him and wonder what happened to her. Is she in rehab? Did she die? Or did another user take her away from him? In a few months, he too is gone.

Kelly and her boyfriend, Tom, still have each other. Tom goes to jail for two weeks, and Kelly tells me how another street friend of theirs suggests that she partner with him. "Not in that way," she says to him. "You know I'm married. I don't tolerate that shit. Just cause I'm nice to you doesn't mean I want to sleep with you." She still gets up her four dollars every four hours and uses, usually in the company of friends, hidden in the bushes beneath Park Terrace. Tom and Kelly always shoot up together. Tom takes his hit first, and after waiting a couple of minutes, to make certain he doesn't slump over and is alert enough to watch her, Kelly injects herself.

While it is good to be paired up, there comes with it a certain codependence. You need someone else to stay safe, but there is no one to talk you into quitting. It is hard for one partner to quit if the other isn't ready to. I think about Sarah Howroyd's story. Sarah is the woman whom I sat across from at the opioid conference. She is a social worker and ex-user who now runs the Heroin/Opioid Prevention and Education Initiative in Manchester, which helps get users into rehab instead of jail. The tale she tells me is chilling.

She grew up in a *Brady Bunch* home, a loving daughter and an A student. The only hint of what lay ahead was when, at age twelve, she got Demerol after a procedure at a children's hospital. She vividly recalls sitting in a wheelchair and saying to her father, "Dad, if this is what it feels like to be drunk, I'm going to get drunk every single day." She goes to school in Boston, gets her degree in social work, and falls in love with an engineering student. One afternoon they have a rear-end crash on the way to Home Depot in Manchester while they are home visiting her sick father. The car in front of them stops suddenly, and the car behind them slams into theirs. They both have neck and back pain and are taken to the emergency department by ambulance, but they are released hours later and told to follow up with their physician back in Boston. Their doctor, Dr. Ellen Malsky, prescribes them each six 20 mg pills of oxycodone per day. This is twelve times a typical starting dose. Sarah follows the directions for a year and a half. Her boyfriend shatters his wrist in an accident. In pain, he takes more of his prescription than he should and even takes some of Sarah's. Sarah's doctor, who, unknown to Sarah, is now under pressure for her prescribing practices, cuts Sarah and her boyfriend off when she realizes he is no longer taking the pills as prescribed. The worst thing you can do to someone on 120 milligrams of oxycodone a day, Sarah says, is cut them off.

To avoid sickness, they start buying pills from friends of friends. They buy one hundred 80 mg oxycodones for $3,400. This lasts them a week. They learn to suck the coating off the pills and scrape them down to a powder so they can snort them. One day, lacking both the money to buy pills and a buyer to supply them, her boyfriend says that all he can find is heroin. She is so sick that she doesn't care. Six months later, in a state of desperate sickness, she agrees to inject for the first time, a practice her boyfriend has already started. She says people set limits on what they are willing to do, or claim to set such limits, but the desperation and the sickness push people beyond them. She says withdrawal is so painful that it even hurts to blink.

Drugs eventually destroy their relationship. Sarah says the drugs, and the stress of trying to avoid being sick, lead to nastiness, rage, and fighting. Addiction brings out sides of a person you couldn't have imagined, she says. She shudders at the thought of how she behaved toward people she loved. In the end, she leaves the man she describes as the love of her life. She doesn't want to die; this is not what she signed up for. She wants to get married someday and have children. She detoxes on her own, is sober for two years, relapses, develops endocarditis, almost dies from it, recovers, and then doesn't use again. She keeps in touch with her ex-boyfriend. There is no loss of love; it is just the drugs that keep them apart. She devotes her time as a social worker to helping other users. She gets a phone call one day with the news—her ex-boyfriend is dead of an overdose. She fights off the urge to use and doesn't relapse despite her deep sadness. She tells other users it gets easier with time. She considers herself one of the lucky ones.

Sarah later finds out that Dr. Malsky, who prescribed them the 120 milligrams of oxycodone a day, was on Purdue Pharma's "Region Zero" list, a secret watch list of top prescribers who, Purdue knew, were prescribing beyond reasonable limits and whom the company nevertheless urged to keep prescribing in high numbers. In the case of Dr. Malsky, the pressure to prescribe persisted, even after one of her patients died of an overdose. When Blue Cross Blue Shield drops Dr. Malsky from its list of approved doctors for her overprescribing, 75 percent of her patients switch their insurance plans to stay with her. Purdue continues to push her to prescribe, until on an office visit, a company representative finds out she's lost her license to practice. Shortly afterward, Dr. Malsky, who told Sarah opioids weren't addictive, commits suicide.[1] Records show that Dr. Malsky prescribed more than 114,000 Purdue pills in her last three years of practice.[2]

When I see a using couple now, I wonder where their loyalties lie? With each other or with the needle?

A young woman is unresponsive in a battered Ford in the Burger King parking lot with agonal respirations. We think the boyfriend called 911, but it might have been a passerby. While the woman is cyanotic, and breathing only four times a minute, she comes to with stimulation, so we decide naloxone is unnecessary. She admits to doing a bundle of heroin, a little more than she usually does. She gave herself a strong dose but hasn't quite overdosed. Lethargy is what she was seeking. I give her a little shake when she starts to nod off. We have a conversation on the way to the hospital. She has been using heroin for years. She is also on methadone, but she missed her daily dose at the dispensary this morning. I ask her how she got started on heroin, and she says she started with prescription opioids following spinal fusion surgery. She got hooked on them, and when she had a hard time getting enough to ease her pain and addiction, heroin was cheaper and easier to find. "Where's my pocketbook?" she asks.

"Your boyfriend has it." The officer on the scene gave it to him. Once the boyfriend knew he wasn't being arrested, I thought he had offered to hold her pocketbook.

"My boyfriend! Why did you give it to him?" She is quite upset: "It's my pocketbook!"

"But he's your boyfriend," I say. "He called 911. He saved your life."

"You can't give him my pocketbook!"

"Why not?" She looks at me like I am a complete fool not to understand.

"We're drug addicts!" she shouts.

She asks again at the hospital about her pocketbook and then asks if her boyfriend is there yet. No sign of him. She starts wailing. She obviously knows him better than I do.

A tall young woman in leopard-print pants, and sporting a hairdo like Ginger's from *Gilligan's Island*, meets us at the apartment door. She is high. Her balance, as she sways in front of us, is so bad that I'm getting dizzy just looking at her. "Thank you for coming so quickly," she says.

"Is he breathing?" I ask.

"Yes, but he won't wake up. He had his methadone dose upped today, and he took some of my benzos. I did CPR on him."

The apartment has hardwood floors, high ceilings, and big windows that look down on the city from the fourth floor of the recently renovated building. I follow her as she stumbles down the hall. "This way."

A muscled, bare-chested, bearded man in his thirties lies on the bed, clearly on the nod but breathing. He has a strong pulse. After some stimulation, he sits up with a jerk to see me, my partner, and four firefighters.

"What did you do?" he says to his girlfriend in a harsh tone.

She begins to cry. "I saved your life," she says. "I did CPR on you. Gave you thirty and one. I threw cold water on you. You almost died." ("Thirty and one" is a ratio of compressions to ventilations in CPR.) She looks at me and says, "Tell him. Tell him I saved his life."

"I don't want to go anywhere. I'm fine," the man says. "This is my house. Get the fuck out."

"You should go to the hospital," I say. "You shouldn't mix benzos with methadone."

"We're both on methadone," she tells me again. "I have a note so that I can take clonidine. I need it for my anxiety. He doesn't normally take it. They upped his dose today, and then he took three of my Klonopins . . . that I know of."

"And he did heroin," Bryan says.

"No, he didn't."

"I found three bags in the bathroom," my partner says. "Sweet Heart." Sweet Heart is a brand making the rounds.

"Hmm," she says, "I'm going to have to rethink this." She says to her boyfriend, "How come you didn't tell me you scored some heroin?"

"It was just four bags," he says.

"I'm hurt."

"I have nothing to say. I just want these people out of here." We try to convince him to go to the hospital. "I know my rights," he says. "I don't have to go. She shouldn't have called you." We argue the fact that he mixed benzos with the heroin on top of the methadone, which makes it necessary for him to be monitored. "You can't make me. You're not going to arrest me, are you?"

"No, we are not the police."

"Good Samaritan, Good Samaritan," the girl says, waving her hands in the air. "You can't arrest us, right?"

"No one is arresting anyone. We just want him to get care." In Connecticut, like many states, there is a Good Samaritan law that protects people who report an overdose from being arrested for their drug use, provided that they don't have outstanding warrants or are selling drugs.

"I gave him thirty and one," she says, "and put cold water on him. I'm an X-ray tech. Tell him not to be mad at me. I saved his life." She turns to him and frowns. "Honey, I love you, even though I'm mad at you. I don't want you to stop breathing again. You need to go."

He lets out his breath and stares straight ahead. "All right," he says, "I'll go. Get me my sandals and my phone. Where's my phone?"

At the hospital, after we leave our patient care report with the nurse, we see the girlfriend has climbed into the bed with the patient. She cuddles him, brushing his hair, while he taps away on his cell phone. "I did thirty and one on you," she purrs in his ear. "You should share with me next time. I saved your life."

Kelly and Tom, along with many others who were living under the highway, get arrested by the Amtrak police for being on Amtrak property. They all get tickets and a date to appear in court. They live now in a small tent in the thicket off Interstate 84 West. In anticipation of winter, which is rapidly approaching, they have a plan to get off drugs and get a room together, which was offered to them by a friend on the condition they stop using. They have gotten some Suboxone and are going to take it one of these days.

Because Suboxone contains a small amount of naloxone, they have to wait until they are in withdrawal to take the Suboxone, or else it will throw them into sudden, strong withdrawal. If they time it right, though, Suboxone will ease their cravings; and if taken for several days, it will help keep them from using while making their detox tolerable. When given under a doctor's care, Suboxone, a form of medication-assisted therapy, can aid people in getting off heroin. I don't want to spoil their plan by telling them that it is important to get therapy at the same time they are taking Suboxone. The combination will help them resist the daily triggers compelling them to use.

We see Kelly one morning, and she is all smiles and walking tall. "I feel great," she says, "no cravings, nothing. I haven't used since last night. I took a Suboxone."

"How's Tom?"

"He's puking in the tent."

"Keep the faith," I say.

At five o'clock that evening, we are across the park when I look up on the hill and see Kelly, Tom, and a few other users enter the tall thicket beneath the road. The next day when we talk, she shrugs: "We just didn't time it right."

Early on a cold morning, before the darkness has completely lifted, we get called for an overdose on the basketball court in the park. My partner pulls out the stretcher, and I sling the big house bag over my right shoulder and carry the heart monitor in my left hand. The fire department responders stand in a semicircle over a body, their breaths visible in the chill. One of the guys gives the finger across the throat sign to say we won't need the stretcher. As I get closer, I see two long legs sticking out from under the blanket. I pull the blanket back and stare at the face. When people die, their soul leaves the body, and their face becomes almost unrecognizable to those who knew them when they were alive. Still, the face is familiar. I strain to recognize her. Then we spot a tattoo on her neck: a faded pony. "That's Janis," a firefighter says. I look at her face again. It is white and waxen. She's been dead for hours. Her limbs are cold and stiff. Her mouth is shut by rigor mortis. Her hair has lost its color. I run my six-second strip of flatline asystole to confirm death. A slow drizzle has started. I pull the blanket back over her face. I wonder who, if anyone, will get a phone call about her. Once the police arrive, we head back to the street, past the empty playground. The morning is black, white, and gray.

Mental Health

Opioid deaths are generally classified as accidental overdoses. In 2017 Massachusetts began reporting opioid deaths as "All Intents," whereas the state previously had reported them as "Unintentional/Undetermined."[1] The state points out that adding suicide deaths increases the count only marginally: merely 2 percent of all opioid deaths in Massachusetts were confirmed suicides.[2]

Connecticut reports opioid deaths under the category of "accidental drug-related" deaths. If a person leaves a suicide note and then injects himself with a lethal amount of heroin, the resulting death would not count in the state's total. In most cases, though, it is hard to determine whether an overdose was a suicide.

An NPR *All Things Considered* broadcast from March 15, 2018, asks, "How Many Opioid Overdoses Are Suicides?" It offers a fairly persuasive argument that the numbers are much higher than reported.[3] The program quotes Dr. Maria Oquendo, past president of the American Psychiatric Association, as saying that the suicide rate could be anywhere from 24 to 45 percent of all opioid deaths.

Should this change the way we view the current crisis? I don't think so. There is a strong link between addiction and mental illness. People use opioids not just because the drug has rewired their brain and elevated a need for opioids above the normal human drives for food, sex, and parenting children; many people also use opioids because they want to escape loneliness, shame, and despair.

Research into addiction suggests that setting and sociality influence drug use. For instance, 90 percent of Americans addicted to heroin in Vietnam were able to kick the habit after returning home. The reason they were able to do so, it has been argued, is because they returned to places where they had a strong support network, a family, and a job that helped them function as members of society.[4]

Other experimental evidence comes from the famous rat park study. Previous studies had shown that rats would ingest drugs until they died. Another researcher noted that the rats in these studies were confined in small cages with no interaction with other rats. This researcher and his colleagues redid the experiment but changed the isolating cages to a rat amusement park, where the animals had food, running wheels, and lots of companionship, including other rats to mate with. Guess what? The rats occupying the park drank far less drug solution than the rats kept in isolation. Even rats that had been in isolation and were addicted stopped ingesting drugs when put in the rat park.[5]

What did that experiment show? Isolation led to addiction, while social interaction helped fend it off. While the study has been criticized as being overly simplistic,[6] there is a lesson from it for us. When we treat users like human garbage and berate them, and then release them from the ED two hours later in withdrawal with instructions to stop using heroin, how can we expect them not to use a drug that temporarily makes them forget about how bad their life has become?

I think that many people addicted to drugs who have fallen to the bottom may not have the strength to climb back up. Some may just give up. Maybe one night, instead of doing five bags of No Evil,

they decide to do ten. Accident or suicide? You can call it unde-
termined. Either way, another human being is lost to us.

Some people use heroin because their life is so haunted that
they cannot stand to face it. Many users have backgrounds of sexual abuse, anxiety, and depression.

William went to the same junior high school I did, although
many years later. I talk to him sometimes when I see him walking up Park Street. He is skittish, but at the same time, I feel that
he wants to talk. He tells me he has been an addict for ten years,
with a couple years off for rehab and recovery before relapsing. He
says he was sexually abused by a teacher, and that has fucked him
up. I google it one day to see if his case made the news, but I can
find no stories. I don't ask for any of the details. I do read about
the link among childhood abuse, post-traumatic stress disorder,
and opioid abuse.[7] I have several patients tell me they were abused
growing up. They talk about having a poor self-image and self-
loathing. I remember years ago hearing this same explanation
from patients and thinking they should just get over it, but I understand now how such an experience can affect the brain.

Vincent lost his wife and baby in a car accident. They were killed
by a drunk driver in Puerto Rico. The driver was from a well-
connected family and was found innocent at trial. On his way out
of the courtroom, he taunted Vincent, who tells me how much he
misses his wife and child. He says he is tired of living like he is.
He says he doesn't use anymore. He just needs money to pay for a
room to sleep in every few nights so that he can get a shower. I see
him in line at the needle exchange van. He pretends not to see me
when I drive by. Sometimes when I drive down Park Street, I see
him sitting in the doorway of a vacant building, no life in his eyes.

DJ got hurt in a motocross accident. His doctor gave him a six-
month prescription for pain pills. One night he came home and

found his girlfriend dead—hanging in his closet. He kept taking the pills so that he didn't have to think about her. That was ten years ago. He tells me he is getting off heroin, as he can't stand to look at himself in the mirror, but when I ask him how and when, he has no plan, no exit strategy. He sits outside McDonald's every day, head down, reading and hoping people hand him some change. Every day he looks worse than the day before; his eyes are dark and hollow.

We respond to an overdose on Babcock Street, in an alley behind a building. Fire first responders arrived before us. A familiar scene. They are hunched over the patient, the Ambu bag out. They have already given her 4 milligrams of Narcan. I stand over them looking at the patient. I can't see her face because the mask obscures it, but I notice that she is tiny. When they lift off the mask for me, I can clearly see it is Veronica. I last saw her a month and a half ago and had wondered what was going on with her. Did she go back to Woodbury to stay with her sister, as she always does when she tries to get clean? Or had she died alone in an alley such as this one? At least I know she is alive. I have the firefighter stop bagging for a moment, and though she is still unresponsive, I notice that her respirations have picked up. The ground is cold, so we lift her up onto our stretcher and then bag her on the way to the ambulance. We load her in the back, and I barely have her hooked up to the capnography to monitor her carbon dioxide when she opens her eyes with a start. She looks at me blankly.

"Veronica," I say.

She tears the capnography cannula out of her nose. She squirms and tries to undo the belts. "No, no," I say.

"Get it out of me! Get it out of me!" she shouts. My partner, who has already started driving to the hospital, asks me if I need a hand.

I am six eight and weigh 230 pounds. My patient is maybe four and a half feet tall and weighs eighty pounds. "No, I'm okay," I say, as I parry the blows and kicks she directs at me.

"Help me! Get it out of me!" she screams.

Two police cars are following us, as is police practice. I can understand it with regular-size people, but this seems unnecessary. I am glad she is so small because I would be in for an ass whupping if she was normal size. She is very, very pissed. The last time I saw her I gave her a big, sweet Cara Cara orange. It was my only one, but I had been glad to see her on the street, to hear how she was doing, and to give her encouragement, and I knew how much she liked oranges. Now, she doesn't seem to recognize me, or if she does, the prior gift has bought me no mercy from her. "Help me!" she screams. "Get it out of me!" By the time we make it to the hospital, she has exhausted herself. She lies on her side panting and then vomits all over herself and the stretcher.

I supported the new 4 mg intranasal naloxone for laypeople and first responders who either don't have an Ambu bag or are not experienced at using one. The 4 mg dosage restores the overdosed person's respirations sooner and helps prevent hypoxic injury. But now it seems that with every overdose call I go on, I get there just in time for the revived person either to try to kick my ass or to vomit on me. Four milligrams administered intranasally, which is the equivalent of 2 milligrams intramuscularly, may just be too much for some people.

I check on Veronica at the hospital several hours later and am glad that she is still there. She looks wiped out and is starkly pale. She tells me that she told the hospital staff she wasn't ready to go back out on the street. I don't blame her because when we brought her in, she didn't have a cent on her. Her purse was empty. And no ID either. Robbed again. She tells me they are going to transfer her to the psych wing because she told them she wanted to kill herself.

"I'm glad you're getting help," I say.

She tells me she had gone to stay with her sister again. As always, though, it lasted about a month before they had enough of each other and she came back to Hartford and started using heroin again. I kid her about how crazy she got when she came around from the Narcan. She smiles and says, "Narcan always makes me crazy."

"Crazy," I say. "You went completely ape on me."

"You didn't have to give me so much Narcan."

"I didn't give it to you; the fire department did. That's the only size they carry. I would have given you only a little; you know that."

"I am always violent when I get the Narcan. I don't react to it well."

"At least you're alive," I say.

She shrugs. The shrug saddens me, as I sense she is truly ambivalent about living or dying.

The next day, I am off from work. My partner texts me to say he's transporting her from the psych wing to a substance abuse facility. I text him in reply, "Tell her I am proud of her."

He texts back later, "She said thank you."

In EMS you always want to know the follow-up, the rest of the story. Will she beat it this time? Can she stay clean? Can she find a new life for herself? Or will I see her walking Park Street again? Hanging with the dealers who like to watch her dance. Will I have to hold an Ambu bag mask over her face again? Or will I or some other medic find her cold and stiff, her spirit long flown away?

I call the time of death on two fatal overdoses in one week. Both men are in their forties. One is in a low-rate motel by the highway. He sits by the window in his breezeless room, the curtains pulled apart just enough for him to see the cars driving past on the highway. His head has rolled back, his mouth open. He is stiff with rigor mortis and surrounded by half-unpacked moving cartons that hold his tattered belongings. The room is dirty. The TV shows video footage of the shootings of police officers in Dallas. The ashtrays overflow with butts. There are scattered glassine envelopes with a monkey stamped on them.

The other man is in the guest bedroom of a small apartment where he is staying with his sister and her four-year-old daughter. He lies back on the neatly made bed, his feet on the floor, his eyes staring at the ceiling, his skin cold and grayish blue. On the wall is a picture of Disney's *Little Mermaid*. On the bureau is his prescription for buprenorphine, a drug to dampen opioid cravings. His sister says he has been clean for three months. She and her daughter spent the night at her mother's and returned in the morning to find him here.

Were these overdoses accidents? Or were these men just tired of what their lives had become? Did they give themselves more heroin than they knew they could handle, choosing to die in the soft cushion of heroin rather than live on in a world too hard for their daily breath and trespass?

Age

When I used to think about the stereotypical heroin user, I pictured a man in his late twenties or early thirties, skinny and tattooed, with track marks on his arms, but I now know that users are of all ages. There are more heroin overdose victims in Hartford over the age of fifty than there are under the age of thirty.[1]

She is a woman of sixty-two years, obese, weighing around 260 pounds; her hair is gray and tied back behind her head in a ponytail; her clothing is threadbare and could use laundering. She has two canes beside her with which she walks slowly and painfully on skinny legs that can barely support her weight. She sits now on a concrete barrier near the bus stop. She fell walking down the avenue, and her leg is killing her: ten out of ten pain. It doesn't help that she's been up doing crack cocaine all night. When my partner asks her about her medical history, she mentions arthritis and cardiac arrest. The cardiac arrest occurred during an overdose earlier in the week at Colt Park in the south end of Hartford. She says her chest is still sore from CPR.

We ask her if she remembers what the bag of heroin she overdosed on looked like. She says it was white—no stamp. She says she bought it from a King gang member who is not her regular dealer. She bought only two bags, and it knocked her out. She says it was white heroin. We show her pictures of some of the bags we have been seeing lately. She nods her head with recognition at some; others she has not seen. She says the unmarked one she got was particularly strong, and there is also a potent batch going around in yellow bags with no markings.

We ask her how a sixty-two-year-old woman from a suburban assisted-living complex came to be buying heroin in Hartford. She says she has bad arthritis, and the medicine her doctor gave her was expensive and, after a while, didn't help. Monte, the maintenance guy at the complex, sometimes sold her Percocets and then offered her heroin. He wanted $10 for a bag. In time, she learned she could get it herself for $5 a bag. A girl with tattoos in her beauty salon gave her a beeper number she could call for a hookup, and she'd take the bus in to meet the man. A $5 bag of heroin was cheaper than $30 for 30 milligrams of Percocet. Of course, she is now homeless (she uses a friend's suburban address to receive mail), has hepatitis C, and sore ribs from the CPR she got on the day she couldn't find her regular dealer and ended up getting white heroin from a Latin King.

I ask her how she knew that she bought it from a King. The Latin Kings used to wear their colors, black and gold, but they have gone somewhat underground now so as not to stand out to law enforcement or the public. Better for business. They still control much of the drug trade in the city. "By the tattoo on his arm," she says, "a lion with a crown. Plus," she adds, "everybody knows the Kings rule the park."

I believe that the number of opioid overdose deaths is underestimated, particularly in the elderly population. If we find a seventy-five-year-old man cold and in rigor mortis in his apartment, with a belt around his bicep, a syringe in his arm, and empty heroin bags on the table next to him, then we can assume it was a heroin overdose. But let's say the man snorted a couple bags of heroin, flushed the empty bags down the toilet, went into the living room, turned on the TV, and then slowly nodded off and stopped breathing. Who would think the seventy-five-year-old man with a history of heart trouble had died of a heroin overdose? We would pronounce him dead. The police would come, call the medical examiner's office, and report nothing suspicious. The medical examiner's office would decline the case, and the funeral home would come and take him away.

Or imagine another scenario. That same seventy-five-year-old man snorts his usual two bags of heroin, which eases the pain in his arthritic knees and puts him in a happy mood. He gets out of his car and walks toward the grocery store. He collapses in the parking lot. One of the bags of Sky High had a hot spot of fentanyl in it. He lies there on the pavement, no longer breathing. Fortunately, we arrive within minutes. I feel a faint pulse in his neck. My partner begins bagging him. I put him on the heart monitor and find him in a strange bradycardia (slow heartbeat). He is maintaining blood pressure, but the twelve-lead electrocardiogram of his heart's electrical impulses is concerning. I am guessing he is having a heart attack or maybe a stroke. His pupils are pinpoint, but he is also lying under the bright sun. His level of exhaled carbon dioxide is 84. The police officer reports that he has an inhaler in his car. I am thinking there may be a respiratory cause for his heart's distress, but his lungs are clear. On a hunch, I give him a little bit of naloxone intravenously, just in case. And, in moments, he is back to breathing on his own, although he is still unresponsive. We load him in the ambulance and transport him with priority to the hospital. When I turn the patient over to the hospital, I admit to the doctor that I don't know what is going on, although I do mention he initially had pinpoint pupils. They are now back to a normal size, but he is also no longer looking up at the sun. When I stop by later to see how he is doing, I am told that his chart shows he has twice before been hospitalized for similar episodes. He has a long history of substance abuse. His sixty-eight-year-old girlfriend arrives and admits that he likes to snort heroin every day.

If he hadn't collapsed in public and gotten medical attention quickly, he could have easily lapsed into asystole at his age, and he would have gotten the standard paramedic treatment of epinephrine doses. And when he didn't respond to that, who would have guessed it was a heroin overdose? It's doubtful the medical examiner would have taken his case, and his body would have been released to the local funeral parlor, his heroin death a secret taken to the grave.

We find a seventy-nine-year-old woman slumped forward in her wheelchair, agonal respirations, pinpoint pupils. If not for the glassine envelope stamped "Dance" on the ground next to her, who would think heroin? A spray of naloxone, and she is back to herself, complaining of her teeth hurting from her recent dental work. Heroin is cheaper than aspirin, she tells us, and works much better.

A man is trembling, sitting on a bed in a motel room near the highway. Sometimes, these rooms are filled with the patient's worldly belongings, but this room seems to have only a bed, dresser, chair, and TV. The man is in his early sixties, a portly man with white hair and liver spots on his hands. A woman in the room with him is of an indeterminate age. She wears a pink tank top and gray yoga pants with flip-flops, even though it is cold and blustery outside. She is the one who called 911. When I say she is of indeterminate age, I mean she could be anywhere from thirty to fifty. She appears to be missing a fair number of teeth, and her arms lack the muscle tone of a younger woman. While he talks to us, she walks behind him and pantomimes shooting up heroin. He says he is a diabetic and hasn't eaten or taken his insulin for a couple of days. He says he got robbed last night and has no money. He is going to have some funds transferred to him tomorrow. We check his sugar, and it is 485. The normal range is 80 to 120, and 485 is in the danger zone. If he doesn't take insulin soon, he could develop diabetic ketoacidosis and go into a coma. We try to persuade him to go with us, and he keeps refusing: "No, no, I'm fine. I'll get some insulin tomorrow. I'm fine, really."

He doesn't look fine. While it would be easy for us to leave, I have done this job long enough to know when someone needs to go to the hospital, so I persist. "Listen," I say. "Look around this room. Do you want to die in this room? You have a couple of hours, and then your mind is going to get really fuzzy. You may fall asleep. In your sleep you'll lapse into a coma. We'll return in the morning to find only your body here because you will have been long gone by then. If the nice lady wakes up beside you, she may notice you've become awfully cold, and we wouldn't want her to have to go through that, would we?"

"You got to go, honey. I'll pay for your insulin," the woman says. "We have to take care of you."

His eyes blink, and he looks from side to side. "Okay," he says, "I'll go."

Outside the room, as we walk him to the stretcher, the woman tugs at my sleeve and says something about his name. I take out a pen and pad and am prepared for her to tell me his name and date of birth. "No, no," she says. "I need to know what his name is. I just met him yesterday. They won't let me see him at the hospital unless I know his name."

Okay then. I get his name for her. She thanks me and says she'll be there in a little while. She sticks her head in the back of the ambulance before we shut the door and says, "Tell them, I'm your granddaughter." Granddaughter, I'm thinking, may be a stretch.

On the way to the hospital, I put in an IV line and start running in fluid. He finally admits to me that he did twenty bags of heroin last night. He says his wife threw him out of his home, and he has been living in the hotel for the past week. I asked him how he got robbed, but he doesn't want to talk about it. I tell him he needs to have Narcan with him if he is going to use heroin. I explain where he can get it. I give the whole rap about not using alone and doing tester shots.

When we get him in his ED room, he is very thankful. He makes eye contact as he shakes our hands. I can tell he is worried about his physical shape. "They'll take good care of you here," I say.

The next Sunday I am working with Andrew Eccles, an EMT whom I will soon begin training to be a paramedic. We are talking about the heroin epidemic, and he tells me he did a DOA (dead on arrival) at the same motel by the highway on Saturday afternoon. Sixty-something man, just released from the hospital. Cops found a syringe and were treating it like a crime scene. They didn't find any heroin bags; they said it looked like the room had been cleaned before they got there, aside from the syringe they found under the bed. The man's wallet was empty. I queried about the room and the patient. It was the same man.

My partner mentions that he found the patient in an odd position—on the ground in a praying position, leaned against the bed. I tell him that this is actually a common position for the body in an opioid overdose death.

A couple of years back I went on a call that really disturbed me. At eleven in the morning at a motel in town, a maid finds the door to one of the rooms unlocked and goes in and screams. We arrive to find a naked man on the floor, his butt up in the air facing us. He is cold, resting on all fours, stiff as can be, his head turned to the side. On the table by the bedstead is a mobile phone, vibrating. I see that it's full of text messages: "Honey, are you okay?"

"Honey, when are you coming home?" "Is everything all right? I am worried."

My partners and I discuss our theories of how he may have died. Based on other evidence in the room, my partners speculate that he may have been having anal sex when he either suffocated or had his neck snapped. We guess his partner noticed he was dead and fled the scene without calling anyone. I run my six-second strip of asystole. Presume him dead.

I keep expecting to see a report of the murder in the paper, but there is nothing. The security footage from the hotel ought to have captured who was there with him. How could anyone leave another human being like that?

Later, I am attending a seminar on death scenes, and I find myself looking at a slide of a dead man's bottom up in the air. The same man. I learn that he died of an opioid overdose. This praying frog position is a common one when people collapse from opioid overdose. We are shown eight more photos of dead people in similar positions; all are opioid deaths.

In my job as EMS coordinator, when I am reading other paramedics' run forms for quality assurance, I come across similar cases. Patient found dead, on knees, face down in the couch. Patient found in bathroom kneeling, face down against toilet, syringe on the floor next to her. My guess is that as the opioid shuts down their breathing, their sight grows dim, and they get suddenly lightheaded. They are just conscious enough to control their fall forward, and then they are out.

I try to picture now the final hours of the man we took to the hospital for high blood sugar. He gets his insulin, gets a wire transfer from his bank, and goes back to the hotel with the woman of indeterminate age. Either she or he buys heroin: a half a stack of fifty bags. Party time. They shoot up. The only problem is that the bags of heroin are laced with fentanyl. One of the bags contains a hot spot, a lethal clump of fentanyl. He injects, and a moment later his breathing slows, his vision goes dark, and he slumps forward to his knees, his arms out before him.

When his acquaintance awakes from her prolonged nod, she sees him there. She gives him a little shake, but he is already gone. She knows this because this is not the first man she has been with who used heroin. She carefully takes the remaining bags of heroin and any paraphernalia. She does not see the syringe that has rolled under the bed. She slips his wallet out of his pocket, takes the remaining bills, and puts the wallet back. She lets herself out into the night.

I wonder if she remembers his name. I wonder how many other people are out there who have been in similar situations, finding a companion dead, robbing his body, and slipping out the door.

It is a brutal world.

The War on Drugs

In 1971, President Richard Nixon started America's War on Drugs that continues today. According to former top aide John Ehrlichman, the entire reason for the war was to target hippies and blacks, who Nixon considered to be his enemies. By associating hippies with marijuana and LSD and blacks with heroin, and criminalizing the possession of both, he could disparage them and attack them with righteousness.[1] The resulting hysteria led to mass incarceration, the spending of untold billions, and little to show for results, as the drug problem in America today is killing more than it ever has. In 2018, law enforcement agencies in the United States made over 1.65 million drug arrests. That's one drug arrest every nineteen seconds.[2] But none of this has slowed the demand or the supply of drugs. And the potency of the drugs is far stronger and, in the case of fentanyl, far more lethal today.

A picture in Hartford's local newspaper shows fifty thousand bags of confiscated heroin, all laid out on a table in neat ten-bag bundles. It seems like a lot of drugs and a cause for celebration, another battle won in the war. But for users with a two-bundle-a-day habit, which amounts to twenty bags daily, fifty thousand bags are a year's supply for just seven users. Despite the bust, users in Hartford won't have to look too far tomorrow to get their fix.

Here is an apocryphal story.

An old man sits on a bench in front of the police substation in one of the worst areas of town. When he sees the narcotics sergeant, he says, "How goes the War on Drugs?" The sergeant says, "Great. We put twenty dealers away this week. Sent them all to prison." The old man sees the sergeant the next week and says, "How goes the War on Drugs?" "Outstanding," the sergeant replies. "We put thirty-seven dealers away this week." This goes on week after week, the number of arrests goes higher and higher. Finally, one day, the sergeant answers the old man, "Best week ever. We put away 178 drug dealers just today alone." The old man laughs and says, "Pretty soon, no more prison cells."

A new legal strategy charges a drug dealer with homicide when one of the dealer's customers fatally overdoses and it can be proven that the customer bought the fatal drug from the dealer. In neighboring Rhode Island, a twenty-five-year-old dealer is convicted of second-degree murder for selling $40 worth of Diesel heroin to a twenty-nine-year-old customer who died four hours later. The dealer is sentenced to twenty years in jail. One way to look at this is to say it sends a message to dealers that they better think twice before selling heroin in Rhode Island. The state is tough on crime and does not tolerate drug dealing.

In a newspaper story about it, the dealer expresses regret: "The actions that I did that day, I never meant to hurt nobody." He apologizes both to the mother of the victim and to his own mother.[3] The story mentions that the victim had just been discharged from drug treatment because her insurance would not cover past thirty days. Having been in treatment, her tolerance was no doubt low, and she likely did the same amount of heroin she used to do before going into treatment. People coming out of treatment are at high risk for a fatal overdose because of their lowered tolerance.

Twelve hundred people died of overdose in Connecticut alone in 2019, up from 357 in 2012. In each of the last three years for which data are available (2016–2018), the national numbers have been in the sixty and seventy thousands with no sign of relenting. I do not consider the convicted drug dealer in Rhode Island an innocent participant, but to me he bears less responsibility for the death than do the heads of pharmaceutical companies who admittedly lied about the addicting properties of their opioid drugs. And let's not forget the responsibility of the Drug Enforcement Administration, which approved the manufacture of millions of kilograms of prescription painkillers that flooded the black market with pills.[4]

In Hartford, a twenty-three-year-old is arrested on federal charges for the distribution of heroin branded "KD" that led to two overdose deaths. The minimum sentence is twenty years.[5] The defendant eventually takes a six-year plea deal.[6] Young people across the country are receiving similar sentences, but the death toll continues to climb.

I wonder how high on the dealer chain these young men were. Did they buy, cut, and package the drug themselves, or were they given the powder by higher-ups and told to sell it and then passed most of the profit up the chain? Of the $40 the twenty-five-year-old in Rhode Island received for that one sale, how much profit did he make? Certainly not profit on the scale of the drug companies. And, clearly, the victim was aware of the risks, although using drugs had compromised her ability to weigh them rationally— something known to the policy makers and insurers who created the system that kicked her out of treatment before she was ready.

Will the twenty-year sentence slow the overdose death rate in Rhode Island? Will dealers move to Hartford, where a similar crime for twice as many deaths incurred a mere six-year federal sentence? We will have to wait and see. I think it is less likely to slow the epidemic than to increase treatment options. If the victim had not been kicked out of treatment because she could not afford it without insurance, she would not have died. If the dealer had decided to work at McDonald's instead of in the drug trade, I think the victim would have simply found someone else to sell her what she craved.

A recent study in the *International Journal of Drug Policy* suggests that new laws charging drug dealers with homicide will have little effect. The forty inmates who were interviewed for the study believe such a law might even have the unintended consequence of deterring people from calling 911 to report an overdose. Many dealers support their own habit by selling to others in their circle. Past research found that 70 percent of state prisoners and 59 percent of federal prisoners arrested for drug trafficking were drug-dependent in the month before they committed their crimes.[7] Knowing that selling to someone who overdoses could lead to imprisonment, one friend might leave an acquaintance overdosed and alone rather than risk summoning help that could lead to a twenty-year prison term.[8]

A chilling footnote to the incarcerations of drug users is that few receive treatment for their addiction while in prison. As I mentioned in chapter 7, inmates get detoxed, but their underlying triggers are not addressed. Worse yet, prisoners who are on methadone or Suboxone when they are incarcerated stop receiving the lifesaving medication when the jail door locks them in. When they get out of prison and return to their old environment, many relapse. With their tolerance down, they have the highest risk of fatal overdose. A study in the *New England Journal of Medicine* found that prisoners in Washington State were twelve times more likely to die in their first two weeks after release than were members of the general population (matched for age, sex, and race), and tellingly the ex-cons were 129 times more likely to die of an overdose.[9]

Bryan and I pull the sheet over another patient. Found by an acquaintance, the man is cold and stiff when we get there. A syringe lies by his side, along with empty glassine envelopes branded "New World." The apartment is spare—a mattress, a table, and a chair. "He just got out of jail," a friend of the dead man says. "I told him to be careful."

We just shake our heads. There was no new world waiting for him when he got out.

Although aggressive in its efforts to jail drug dealers, Rhode Island, to its credit, screens all prisoners for opioid use disorder, provides them buprenorphine or methadone, and, upon release from incarceration, provides them with a referral to community-based treatment programs. The state was able to decrease deaths among recently released inmates by an astonishing 61 percent.[10] According to an article in the New York Times, the Bureau of Justice Assistance reported that, in 2017, fewer than 30 of the nation's 5,100 correctional facilities provide methadone or buprenorphine to their inmates. In Connecticut, where 75 percent of inmates have a substance use problem, only two of fifteen facilities provide methadone to patients, even to those who are on long-term methadone when they go to jail. This is the situation, despite the advocacy of Connecticut's state corrections medical director, Dr. Kathleen Maurer. She tells the Times, "We don't take away people's insulin or their asthma inhalers. Why should we take away their methadone?"[11]

Among Connecticut's inmates, Kelly is lucky. When she is sent to the state women's prison in Niantic for two weeks for failing to appear in court for her trespassing charge, she is given methadone daily to keep her from feeling sick, and she is referred to a Suboxone program upon discharge. But when she gets out, she is still homeless and hanging out with her old heroin-using friends. While I welcome her back from her absence, the syringe stuck in her bra tells the story. She shrugs and says, "I don't have to get up as much money now. I'm only using half a bag at a time."

I think if only I had a magic wand that could undo events from the past. I would go back in time to when Kelly's mother offered her that first pain pill or to the time she did heroin by mistake when she misheard *coke* for *dope* from a guy at a party. I would end over-prescription, get the government to crack down on false advertising, and limit the supply. I could end the War on Drugs before it began. I could get people to recognize the problem as medical and not criminal. I could stop the deaths.

But there is no magic wand. All that we have are people's best efforts. There are people like Mark Jenkins, who is dedicated to each user he encounters, determined to do his best to help others. There are people like Sarah Howroyd, who manages to get an appointment with Chief Marc Montminy of the Manchester Police Department. When he tells her his department is arresting as many drug users and drug dealers as possible, she asks him, "How's that working out for you?"[12]

Sarah suggests that the department look at a project started in Gloucester, Massachusetts, where anyone addicted to drugs can walk into the town police station and ask for help. Instead of being jailed, the user is taken to the local hospital, where she's paired with a volunteer who will help her through the treatment process. As the Gloucester police website says, "If you have drugs or drug paraphernalia on you, we will dispose of it for you. You will not be arrested. You will not be charged with a crime. You will not be jailed. All you have to do is come to the police station and ask for help. We are here to do just that."[13]

Montminy tells Sarah that, if she is willing to do the legwork, she will have all his support. The two hit it off and set out creating their own program, the Heroin/Opioid Prevention and Education Initiative. They partner with the Eastern Connecticut Health Network in Manchester and Saint Francis Medical Center in Hartford to get users into treatment and keep them out of jail. Their program becomes a model for others in the state.

We all hope the tide will turn. I see it every day on the streets of Hartford. Police show up at the scene of a patient who has just been revived from an overdose and is now agitated, vomiting, and telling us all off. Instead of throwing him up against a wall and handcuffing him, police officers, in most instances, hold their hands up in a gesture of peace: "You're not in trouble. We're here to get you help. Let the medic examine you. You're not under arrest. We just want you to be safe."

Temptation

I am walking around one morning behind the Dunkin' Donuts plaza on Albany Avenue. In the rear parking lot, there are some trees against a fence, and in between the trees and the fence is a small area where users often shoot up. I check the area every morning, and if no one is sleeping under the trees, I pick up the used syringes and check the empty heroin bags for new brands. On this morning, I notice a thick square of white by the curb. I reach down and see heroin bags with a rubber band around them. It is a bundle of heroin. I have found bundles twice before, but all of the bags were empty. This time, it has a slightly heavier feel. I undo the rubber band and unfold the first bag on top. Holding it up to the light, I can see there is some substance in the bottom of the bag. My goodness. It is heroin. Ten bags, each with 0.1 gram of powdered illegal opioid. The bags are stamped "Tunnel Vision." Someone has dropped it. It is worth $30. I take out a plastic spoon and empty the contents of one bag. A white-brownish powder comes out. It is an amazingly small amount of powder, not enough even to cover the bottom of the spoon. I imagine myself as Telly Savalas in the role of Kojack, the hard-boiled New York City police detective in the old CBS TV show.

I touch my finger to the powder and then touch it to my tongue. It tastes bitter. Yeah, that's heroin. I marvel at the powder and think about putting some up my nose. Just a little. How would I feel? Maybe that little bit might be a clump of fentanyl, and I will keel over dead. I imagine the headline: Paramedic dies of heroin overdose on the job. Or maybe I will feel suddenly great. Truly awesome! Wrapped in the warmth of the gods. Maybe in six months, I will be homeless myself and shivering under these same trees in the rain, waiting to meet my dealer to buy a single bag of heroin to keep the sickness away. Instead, I blow the powder into the wind. I toss the rest of the bags back under the trees.

Later in the day, I wonder whether I should have kept a single bag. I imagine sitting at my desk with the bag of heroin on the table next to an already rigged Narcan atomizer. Simultaneously with snorting the heroin, I will squirt the antidote in my other nostril. In the minute or two before the naloxone takes effect, I will understand what all the fixation is about. I will meet the notorious dragon.

It is just a daydream. I have a wife, kids, and a job I love. Unlike in my youth, when I experimented with many recreational drugs except for heroin—marijuana, amphetamines, cocaine, LSD, and peyote—today I am content with a cold glass of water at the end of the day. Heroin seems to me anything but recreational. For those addicted, it is a full-time job. I am glad that pain pills weren't around in my youth in the circles I traveled in.

A few months later, I am eating roast duck from the A Dong grocery store. A Dong is an awesome Chinese grocery store that has cooked ducks strung up by their heads, fried boar's head, pig's feet, and other delicacies you don't find in other supermarkets. I buy half a duck, which a woman in an apron chops into twelve pieces with a giant butcher's cleaver. To get the meat out from between the bones, I need to use my front teeth. The duck is delicious. Then I hear a snap and feel something wrong in my mouth.

When I was a boy, I went over the handlebars of my bike and was knocked unconscious. I needed an overnight stay in the hospital and many stitches, including some to my upper lip. A few years later, when my adult front teeth should have descended, only one did. The second one must have come out in the accident. I had a fake tooth on a plate for a number of years and then eventually got a bridge, for which they drilled two teeth to nubs and then hung the three-tooth bridge between them. That lasted for many years, until now. Looking in the mirror, I see a man with huge gap in his front teeth.

I go to the dentist and a few weeks later end up in an oral surgeon's chair, where he injects me with Novocain and then drills a hole in the roof of my mouth where he will sink an implant. I can feel nothing except my body and the chair rattling as he drills. When I leave, the receptionist asks me if I want strong pain medicine. Yes, I say, excited. I am about to be prescribed legal pain pills. It is not that I want to start down the road to heroin addiction; it is that I want to have a firsthand experience of what the opening steps might be like. Thanks to provider education and new laws limiting initial prescriptions, I get only eleven Vicodins. Gone are the days of the six-month supply.

That night I am in serious pain. I contemplate taking a pill. I contemplate splitting it in two and taking only half. What if suddenly I am in nirvana? Will this be the beginning of the end? Should I have Narcan at my side in case something goes wrong? I ponder. But my mouth really hurts. I pop a whole pill. Down the hatch.

It turns out to be a letdown. It does ease the pain. I don't feel any queasiness, as some people report, but I certainly don't have the greatest feeling ever. At least I sleep through the night, which at my age is a blessing.

A couple of days later, the pain is gone. I try another experiment. I take only half a pill in the evening. I feel relaxed but nothing special; again, I sleep through the night. I have six and a half pills left. I know I am supposed to throw them away if I don't use them, but I keep them. The hole in my mouth gets infected, and the bone graft doesn't take. So I end up having to get two more holes drilled, but these are less painful. This time they don't offer me a new prescription. Just take Motrin, the doctor says. I know I could ask for opioids, but I don't because I don't need them.

Then one night a few weeks later, I take a whole pill just to take it. I go to bed. I am not certain if it is a dream I am having or the pill I've taken, but I am euphoric in a way I have not been in years. I feel great, like I have no worries and life is good. And, again, I sleep through the night. Praise be. I tell Kelly about the euphoria, and she says that's what happens when you take it just for pleasure.

A few months later, I have a health scare that panics me. I try to imagine what it will mean for my future and my family. I am irritable and have difficulty concentrating. I take a Vicodin, and it chills me out. I sleep through the night, and in the morning, I realize that I am actually not facing all I feared and that, at least for now, everything is okay. It makes me understand just how powerful an opioid can be in blocking emotion and in helping a person cope with what may seem overwhelming.

I have four and a half pills left, but I haven't taken any more. Still, I could see how, if my life sucked and I was in need of feeling better and escaping, there could be magic in that bottle.

I share my experiences with a doctor friend. He tells me that he had a terrible childhood, and then one day, when he was sixteen, he smoked marijuana for the first time and felt happy, truly happy, like the emptiness in him had been filled with warmth. He smoked like a fiend for years. He is glad he never tried heroin; it wasn't in his social circle. He was only able to stop smoking marijuana when he was confronted with a choice: continue heading down the same path or get serious about his life and do something with it. With the right influences at the right time, he was able to get it together.

Years later, he hurts his back and goes to the ED, where a doctor friend gives him a blast of Dilaudid intravenously. *Whoa!* All his pain and all his worries go away, and he feels fantastic. He is thirty-seven years old then, with a wife and family. He knows enough from his job not to seek that feeling again, recognizing it for the demon it is, but he tells me, "If I was seventeen and tried heroin and felt like I did on Dilaudid, I would do anything in the world to find that feeling again." He told his kids not to do drugs until they are at least twenty-one. He doesn't want them doing drugs at all, but he pleaded with them not to take them when their brain is still forming. I tell my kids the same.

Children

Many years ago, R. J. Reynolds tobacco company got into trouble with its Joe Camel advertising campaign, which featured a cool cartoon camel in human clothing who liked to smoke. The campaign was controversial because it seemed to target kids. The American Medical Association tried to get the company to shut down the Joe Camel campaign after a study showed that as many six-year-olds knew that Joe Camel was associated with cigarettes as knew that Mickey Mouse was associated with Disney.[1] Sales statistics indicated a huge increase in underage (twelve-year-olds to seventeen-year-olds) sales of Camel cigarettes, from 0.5 percent of the market to 32.8 percent. Company documents were made public that revealed R. J. Reynolds was indeed targeting kids. Finally, in 1997, the company terminated the campaign and settled a lawsuit by agreeing to donate $10 million to efforts to prevent teen smoking.[2]

The heroin industry in Hartford seems to be taking a similar tack these days, and it is quite disconcerting. Among the brands to hit the streets in recent weeks are Bugs Bunny, Hello Kitty, Dino Babies, and Smurfs, to go along with the previously issued Casper, the friendly ghost.

Spring is here, and the city parks are littered with heroin bags. The users sit on park benches and tear the bags open and snort the fine powder, or they go down to the pavilion by the pond and squat against the brick pillars. There, they fill a 1 cc syringe with heroin solution, tie a USB cord around their arm, and hit any vein they can find that is not sclerosed (hardened) or ulcered. The bags, forgotten, are carried on the wind. Sometimes users seek the privacy of a portable toilet, and a daily check of these toilets reveals the latest brands, the bags having been cast onto the floor or tossed into the urinal.

I watch a six-year-old run across the playground and enter a portable toilet. I wonder what she will do when she sees the bag with Bugs Bunny on it. Will she pick it up? If there are a few grains of powder in it, will she taste it? Or has her mother already warned her? Stay away from those bags. Don't pick up any syringes. Don't talk to strangers.

But this is the world we live in, and I think we need to set some ground rules. I propose that we call all the heroin dealers together for a powwow in the park. No cops. Listen here, we will say. It is not our business to arrest you and put you behind bars—that's a job for the police. But you need to show some respect for our community. If you want to name your product Strike Dead, Killing Time, or Biohazard, go right ahead. If you call it Nightmare on Elm Street, The Purge, or Friday the 13th, be our guest. If you dub it Cobra, Scorpion, or Black Widow, have at it. But Hello Kitty is out of bounds. Same deal with Bugs Bunny, Foghorn Leghorn, Kermit the Frog, and Barney. Got it?

And while we are it, here are some other rules to think about, if you have any decency.

Stop putting fentanyl into brown powder. The folks who don't want fentanyl are staying away from the white powder because fentanyl is white and they don't want to die. You pretend to sell them fine brown powder by spiking it with fentanyl; shame on you.

You already got them addicted; they have to have their hits, so at least let them have the option to avoid sudden death. Danger seekers can continue to run a risk with white heroin, but please let there be some boundaries to your deviousness.

If you are going to sell carfentanil, you can only brand it as follows: "Beware . . . Carfentanil, Elephant Killer, or Lifetime Supply." In this case, *lifetime supply* means one bag and you're dead.

Offer Narcan to all your customers, or offer them a safe place where they can shoot up under the watchful eyes of one of your men. If they overdose, your guy can give them Narcan and call 911. In our state there is no liability for calling 911 for an overdose, unless you are selling drugs at the scene. Get a lawyer to create a shell company or something so that the place where users overdose is not affiliated with your drug dealing business.

On the back of each envelope you sell, stamp this number: 1-800-563-4086. It's the Connecticut Opioid Hotline. If someone calls that number, she will be connected to the closest walk-in assessment center, where she will be evaluated, and the center will try to find the best form of treatment for her and help her with insurance if needed. There are seven assessment centers in the city of Hartford alone.

Our society created many addicts through poor policy that led to the widespread availability of painkillers. Addicts need to get their fix somewhere, until they are ready to get clean. We recognize that drug dealers are filling a demand. If you are going to deal, at least be responsible about it. And, of course, none of this will exempt you from police enforcement of state and federal drug laws.

These ideas may not be that far-fetched. Alixe Dittmore, a programs manager with AIDS Connecticut, who helps run the needle exchange van, tells me of a drug dealer who comes to the van for naloxone and learns how to counsel his users on safe-injection techniques. If he sells to a new customer and knows he has a strong batch, he will insist that the customer inhale a bag in front of him so that he can determine that customer's tolerance. If we are going to commit to harm reduction, we need to enroll all possible assistance. Yes, even drug dealers can help end avoidable deaths.

I ask Kelly about her dealers. She has a few she trusts. I don't want to know who they are, but I am curious about how they interact. She says her main dealer likes her and cuts her breaks. He warns her when the batch may be on the strong side. I get the sense that he gets the same kick out of her that I do. She can be feisty and outspoken. I tell her to do me a favor and talk to her dealer for me. Tell him to spread the word. No more cartoon characters. Stick with skulls. She agrees. "Bugs Bunny is totally inappropriate," she says. "Someone has to look out for the kids."

"We're all in agreement on that," I say. "Talk to him; tell him I said so. Tell him the tall paramedic who walks in the park wants dealers to stop using cartoon characters."

"I'll tell him," she says. "It isn't right. It's not like it's going to hurt his business too much, and he shouldn't be selling to kids."

When I see Kelly next, I ask her how the conversation went.

"Huh?" she says.

"You know, telling the dealers to not use Hello Kitty."

"Oh, sorry, I forgot to. I'll tell him next time."

I just shake my head.

Curiously enough, the next year, aside from the Tasmanian Devil "Back Off" bags, I find only a few bags stamped with a cartoon character, while the city is besieged by bags with skulls on them. Maybe someone somewhere recognized the need for limits.

Community Naloxone

Narcan is readily available in Connecticut. You can walk into nearly any pharmacy in the state, and the pharmacist, provided that the pharmacist has completed the necessary training, will write you a prescription and dispense naloxone to you on the spot, as well as provide a short training session. If you have insurance, the cost is little or nothing. You can also get naloxone for free at the needle exchange van or by attending one of Mark Jenkins's free Thursday night naloxone trainings. Naloxone is all over Hartford.

We get called for an overdose at the bus stop, someone who's possibly not breathing. We arrive in minutes. A man sits on a bench, leaning forward, head down. We approach. I can see his chest is moving. Maybe four times a minute. I give him a shake. He responds slowly. His pupils are pinpoint. I recognize him as a regular on Park Street. His face is very pale. I see some beads of sweat on his forehead.

"Hey, are you all right?"

"Yeah, yeah, I'm fine," he says. I give him another shake. He is breathing better now.

"How much did you do?" I ask.

"I didn't do anything. I'm good. I'm good." He stands and looks around the street. "I'm just . . . I'm just tired, that's all."

"You know what day it is?"

"Monday," he says. Good guess.

"Who's president?"

"Trump."

We let him walk off. He crosses the street and then pukes in the bushes. I walk over to him and ask him again if he is all right. He says he is good and waves me off. He continues to walk off down a side street.

"What was up with him?" my partner asks.

"I don't know. It was like I gave him Narcan, but I didn't."

"Maybe he had an anticipatory reaction to the sirens."

"Maybe."

The next week, we get called to Broad and Grand for an overdose. This is prime OD land. We arrive to find the cops looking around. A man stands against the building and looks a little wobbly. But neither he nor anyone else standing around has anything to say. The call originated from a bodega. The cops go inside and ask. The caller comes out and points to the dumpster. He was right there.

No one is there. The cops think it might be the wobbly guy, but he denies it as he turns and wobbles off. A mystery, but not uncommon of late. Dispatched for an overdose, we clear the scene as unfounded. Another time we are dispatched for an overdose in a portable toilet at a local park. No one is around, and the toilet is empty. In the urinal, we find a single empty vial of Narcan.

I give a talk on the opioid crisis at a paramedic refresher course. One of the medics asks, "Anyone else showing up on calls to find the patient already Narcaned?" There is a chorus of "yeah" and "me too" responses. Could it be that someone has taken it upon himself to patrol the streets? He spots an overdose victim, delivers a squirt or two up the victim's nose, and then disappears. Does he work alone? Or is he but one of an informal corps? Is he unique to Hartford, or does someone like him live in every city beset by the opioid crisis? How many lives has he saved? How many ODs has he reversed? Urban legend or real-life superhero? We joke about a Marvel Comics movie about his life called *Narcan Man*. I can see the theatrical poster featuring a homeless man with a confident smile and a gold tooth, wearing bandoliers of naloxone.

Later I learn of another comic book by the author of the *Lil' Dope Fiend Overdose Prevention Guide*. This one is called *Narcan Saves Lives!* and features Narcania.[1] In the eight-page mini-comic, Narcania, an attractive young woman in a cape, explains how Narcan works and what to do and what not to do during an overdose. She uses her opioid-blocking powers to save Lil' Sallie, who has overdosed for one or more reasons: having low tolerance, using too much heroin or heroin that's too strong, mixing her drugs, or using by herself. Narcania tells the personified figure Death that he'll have to wait. Death says that he sees he's not wanted, and Lil' Sallie thanks Narcania. The comic concludes by telling readers how they can get Narcan and declares, "It should be legal to own and carry it everywhere in America . . . & the World!"

In San Francisco there is a mural named *Narcania vs. Death*, in which Narcania defeats Death with a superhero POW! and saves Lil' Sallie, who declares, "I don't know if there's anything worth living for, but at least I'll get the chance to Find Out!"[2]

Local harm reduction programs in Hartford estimate that their clients have been involved in hundreds of overdose reversals. Alixe Dittmore, who now works for Mark Jenkins, gives out two Narcan kits at a time to certain users who report reversing multiple overdoses. She thinks it is possible for laypeople to reverse more overdoses than EMS, and while users are instructed to call 911 when they give someone naloxone, clearly not all do. Some don't have a phone; others have a fear of police contact. As soon as the victim is breathing again, they split. No need to have cops there to check on any outstanding warrant, which most of them have because an opioid habit precludes their sitting in a courtroom all day waiting to be called for their trespassing or panhandling case. It would not surprise me if Alixe's hunch were right.

There is an anxious crowd on the corner of Hungerford as we come down Park Street with lights and siren going. A woman with tattooed arms waves for us to hurry. A man is on the ground with a crowd clustered around him. I can see another man kneeling, bent over the chest of the fallen man. His arms are together like he is doing CPR. "They hit him twice," a bystander says to me. "Lot of people packing it on this corner."

"He was just walking along and down he went," another says.

"He gave him four in the right," the first man says, and then nodding toward a shorter man wearing a Pittsburgh Pirates hat, he adds, "and he gave him two in the left." The man on the ground opens his eyes and looks around as the crowd cheers.

"You OD'd, man," a rescuer says to him, still holding the syringe with the atomizer on it.

"I did not," he says. "What are you all looking at?"

"Man, you were out. I Narcaned you, fool! And that dude did CPR on you!"

"No, I'm fine," he says. "I just fell out."

"No, man," says the dude with the 4 mg nasal spray in his hand. "You weren't breathing. We gave you Narcan, man."

"No, I'm good. I'm good."

He insists he did not do drugs, but with the crowd's backing, we get him on our stretcher and take him to the hospital. On the way there, he admits to snorting a bag. This is the second time this week he has overdosed, he says.

In Tombstone in the old West, a man would drop a glass in a saloon, and everyone would whip out their six-shooter and point it at him. In Hartford these days, it seems that everyone is also packing. A man drops in the street, and everyone whips out their Narcan.

Does access to naloxone influence an opioid user's decision to use? Some people say it does. That is the crux of a preprint, "The Moral Hazard of Lifesaving Innovations: Naloxone Access, Opioid Abuse, and Crime," which argues that increasing access to naloxone permits risky behavior, unintentionally increases opioid abuse, leads to more crime, and may increase the death rate.[3]

The paper has generated a great deal of controversy. The coauthors assume that naloxone creates a safety net that encourages opioid use because users know they can be revived if they overdose. The coauthors cite evidence for this: a legislator who, at a congressional hearing, said, "Kids are having opioid parties with no fear of overdose"; news reports of police finding naloxone at overdose scenes; and an Ohio police officer who is quoted as saying, "We've Narcan'd the same guy 20 times." The coauthors say their data prove these anecdotes represent valid concerns, even if the anecdote about Narcan parties seems to have little validity.

Other research papers have found the opposite. A paper published in the journal *Addictive Behaviors* shows a small decrease in heroin use among users who underwent naloxone training.[4] A paper published in *Addiction*, which reviews twenty-two naloxone studies, finds that naloxone training programs reduced overall mortality among those trained.[5]

The authors of the "Moral Hazard" paper use the concept of moral hazard, which comes from economics; it means that people may take more risks when they know that others will deal with the consequences. The term gets applied often to insurance. If you have car insurance, you may drive with less care than someone driving without insurance, who would have to bear the full cost of an accident. In the context of the opioid crisis, a user doesn't have to worry about overdosing because a drug is available to revive her. Consequently, she will use more than she would have otherwise. I have doubts that this risk-reward thought process applies well to addicted individuals, who no longer reason effectively when it comes to risk on account of their altered brain chemistry.

As a paramedic with experience dealing with opioid users, and as a member of an overdose working group that seeks to increase access to naloxone, I can say the following.

Users are going to use. I don't think they are going to put off their next hit just because they are out of Narcan and have no one to call 911 if they keel over. Users hate naloxone. They may keep it around to save their or others' lives if they have to, but no one is deliberately getting "Narcaned."

It is true that, by keeping users alive, naloxone allows users to use again. Their survival and continued need for opioid mean that users may commit more crimes to support their habit. That is a trade-off I am willing to make as a human being. No one has ever said that naloxone is the key to ending the epidemic. Naloxone is about keeping people alive until they are ready to get help. I agree with the harm reduction community: dead people can't recover.

We respond to a dispatch for an unconscious man. When I arrive at a second-floor apartment and am directed down a hallway, I hear someone say the man has a pacemaker. I find the man lying on his side on a mattress in the living room. His head is bluish purple. He has vomit on the side of his mouth and pillow. He is not breathing. I feel for a pulse on his thick neck but feel nothing. We begin CPR. Thirty seconds later, the man gives an agonal gasp. We stop CPR. Still no breathing or pulse. The monitor shows a low-voltage heart rhythm. More CPR. A few more agonal breaths.

I have the Narcan out. Narcan has no role for someone in cardiac arrest, but I am not certain he is in arrest; I just can't feel his pulse. If he is in arrest, it won't help, but if he has an impalpable pulse, it could restore his respiratory drive.

I decide to put a needle on the Narcan and give him an intramuscular injection. More compressions, more agonal breaths, and then, at last, a pulse. His carbon dioxide level is 87. We keep bagging him. Soon it drops down to around 40. Two minutes later, he starts moving his extremities and opens his eyes. He is sweaty; his hands are shaking. The good news is that he is back among the living; the bad news is that the high dose I gave him has put him into withdrawal.

When he is coherent enough to speak, he admits to snorting ten bags of heroin. I find the torn empty bags branded "Cobra" stuffed in a small cardboard box with his cigarettes. He has been out of rehab for a week, and this is the first time he has used. He just felt like it, he says. I ask him how he got started. He says he has been using for three years. There was so much heroin in the neighborhood, he thought he'd try it. He is my age: fifty-eight.

I tell him that if he uses after not using for a while, his tolerance is going to be low. I tell him he should never use alone, and when his tolerance is down, he needs to use less. He nods. I tell him where to get Narcan. The needle exchange van will give him free Narcan and train him on how to use it.

There are four or five other people standing in the room now, surprised that their friend is up and talking. "You need to have Narcan," I tell them.

"I have Narcan," says the woman who called 911.

"Why didn't you give it to him?"

"I thought it was his heart. He didn't tell us he was using."

"Well, at least you called 911," I say.

"He could have told us he had some heroin," she says, looking at him disdainfully.

"Next time, tell them," I say to the man, "or at least lay some Narcan by your pillow so they'll get the hint."

"We give you a place to stay, and you hold out on us," she says, shaking her head.

People getting out of rehab, people getting out of jail, or people ending a period of self-imposed abstinence are at the highest risk of suffering a fatal overdose. In Connecticut, prisoners are all given Narcan when they get out of a state prison. I am guessing that people leaving a substance abuse treatment facility are told that, if they use again, they should take a tester shot, start small, and work their way up. Perhaps, though, they are told nothing about using again since they have just graduated from rehab. Maybe optimism should be tempered with realism in this situation. Because relapse rates are high, treatment graduates could well benefit from receiving Narcan too.

I tell users all the time never to do opioids alone, but getting someone to do it with you means sharing, and users may want to keep for themselves what they worked hard to get.

I am called to an overdose. I ask the woman who flagged me down if the patient is still breathing as I get my gear from the side door. The woman says she doesn't know. They hadn't seen him for a week, so they went in his apartment and found him. "Third floor," she says. "He's not moving."

I can smell the body as I go up the stairs toward the rented room. Like each of the last three overdose calls I have been on, the room is spare. He has been dead for a while. Next to his cold body, mottled purple and white, are two unopened packages of the new Narcan nasal spray. He got the message about having Narcan out but must have ignored the "Don't do heroin alone" instruction. I find paperwork that says he was given naloxone when he was discharged from rehab in late November. It looks like someone may have taken one Narcan applicator out of the box but did not open it. Clearly, his neighbors arrived too late to save him. There are no drugs in the man's apartment and no money in his wallet.

I have seen heat maps showing where the overdoses in Hartford are, and these maps square with what I have seen on calls. We map overdoses so that we know where to direct EMS resources. The needle exchange vans are close to two hot spots. Alixe Dittmore sets up an outreach shop for an hour and half each afternoon at the Fastrack municipal bus stop, the site of multiple overdoses and the place where many coming in from the suburbs to buy drugs enter and exit the city. The police certainly do their job of trying to get product off the street, and each week we see pictures in the newspaper of guns, cash, and heroin bags spread out on a table for a bust shot. But people keep dying, and heroin and fentanyl are as prevalent as ever.

Do we leaflet the area? Do we stand on the corner and make public speeches about the horrors of opioids? Maybe we should lease a giant billboard. Instead of it saying, "Just say NO to Drugs," the billboard could say this instead: "There is a lot of bad dope out there that may kill you. Always do a tester shot first. Try not to use alone. If you have just gotten out of rehab or jail, your tolerance is low. Just do a little to start. Have Narcan available. Call 911. You won't be arrested. Your life has value. Stay safe. Please stay safe."

Safe-Injection Site

It is pitch dark, six in the morning in the middle of winter, a day after a large snowstorm. We get called for an overdose on the sidewalk of Hungerford Street. The address is not a surprise—Hungerford is a side road that runs into Park, one block east of Broad. When we arrive, we find no one. We are about to leave the scene when a police officer who has also responded finds a backpack in the snow. A moment later, a man comes down the street to claim the backpack. He seems somewhat confused. One side of him is dripping wet, as though he has been lying in the snow.

"Why are your clothes soaking wet?" I ask.

He hesitates a moment: "I was helping a friend shovel snow." His answer makes no sense. It is six in the morning, and the snowstorm was the day before, ending well before noon.

"We were called for an overdose. Would you know anything about that?"

"Ah, no. I don't use drugs."

"Have you used in the last couple hours?"

"Ohhh, nooo," he says. "Well, maybe seven years ago but not for a long time."

I am skeptical, but he knows the date and his name. "Why don't we take you to Hartford Hospital," I suggest. "You can get your clothes dried out, get something to eat, and maybe even get a checkup."

"No, thank you," he says. "I'll just be on my way." He picks up his bag and heads up the street toward Park.

The cop and I exchange some small talk, and then, as I start toward the ambulance, I see something on the sidewalk. I reach down and pick it up. It is a retainer with three false teeth on it. I can't think of whose it could be except the half-wet guy with the backpack. I start down the street to see if I can catch up to him. "Hey!" I call. "Hey, dude!" It is still pitch black, and I am hurrying down an icy street holding some guy's false teeth. Another uncanny EMS moment, I think. All part of the job. I finally catch up to him.

"Oh, yeah," he says, "I was missing those." He puts them in his mouth. "Thanks."

"You sure you don't want to go to the hospital?"

"No, I'm good." He continues down Park Street, and I head back to the ambulance.

About a half hour later, another ambulance crew gets called for a man in the snow on a street several blocks away. It turns out to be a cardiac arrest. I listen to their radio patch into the hospital. The man is the same age as my patient. I hear them say they gave him Narcan to no effect.

I talk to the crew later and am relieved to learn their man had a brown coat whereas my guy's coat was black. I always worry when a patient refuses transport, or when a patient walks away, that something will happen to him because he didn't go to the hospital. Whenever I hear on our radio the same address that I cleared half an hour before, I worry that I failed to note something important or should have insisted harder that the patient go to the hospital. I ask the medic if he saw any heroin paraphernalia or bags at the scene. He says no, but the man did have fresh track marks, and the hospital said he was a known user. The man was asystole on their arrival. They got a heart rhythm again on the monitor after giving him some epinephrine, but there was no pulse. He was officially pronounced dead at the hospital. It was odd that he died in a snowbank, they remark. I am thinking the same thing. What are the odds of two guys overdosing in a snowbank on a dark Sunday morning? In the summertime, having two guys overdose on a sidewalk within a couple of blocks of each other is not odd at all, but in the winter, in the dark of predawn, it's strange.

Their patient is the second fatality of the morning after an ambulance crew from the south end presumes a man dead who was found by his family in the bathroom with a needle still stuck in his arm. He is cold and has rigor mortis when the crew gets there—long gone. The number of ODs ebbs and flows in the city, but for the last couple of days, they have been on the high end. It is hard to say whether it is a bad batch or the same old kill-you-anyway stuff that is usually sold on the streets of Hartford.

I thought that running down the street and shouting "Dude, your teeth!" might have been the end of my tale, but a month later I learn, as radio commentator Paul Harvey used to say, the rest of the story.

I am taking a man from the jail to the hospital for chest pain. He checks out fine, and we end up talking about the heroin trade. I ask him what the strong brands are, and I am a bit upset when the two brands he names as the most potent—Star Wars and The Finals—I have yet to encounter in my searches for empty heroin bags. They are both by far and away the only bags worth getting in Hartford, he says. And then he tells me a story to illustrate the strength of the brands. A month ago, he says, he was working in a heroin house on Hungerford Street. A heroin house, he tells me, is a place where people can go to buy their heroin ($4 to $5 a bag), a clean needle ($2), and they can shoot up right there under the watchful eyes of house workers. (I did not ask if there was a house fee or a fee for when a house worker helps a patron find a vein.) When users are done, they are free to be on their way, safe in the knowledge they have no heroin or heroin paraphernalia in their possession. And if they overdose while in the house, the house workers have Narcan to revive them. Not a bad business model, I think.

Except, it turns out, the workers are not the most reliable people.

In other countries, there are safe-injection sites overseen by medical professionals who not only protect users against dying from overdose but are also there to help guide them to rehab if they are ready. Such sites are also being considered by some states in the United States. In this Hartford heroin house, however, the staff are users themselves paid in heroin.

The man relates that when The Finals and Star Wars first came out—he admits they are from the same batch, only stamped with different brands—three people overdosed. The guy who was supposed to be watching over them at the heroin house was talking to his girlfriend on his cell phone and stepped out into the hallway, where they had a lengthy argument over the phone. Aware of the potency of the brands, my passenger checked in the watcher's room and saw three people in there, all overdosed, including one who was blue and seizing. He struggled to give them all Narcan. The directions on the box were not easy to understand, he says, but he finally managed to assemble the atomizer and squirted mist in their noses. One of the men came around and proceeded to vomit on the floor. The other two weren't coming around. "We have to call 911," he said to the house supervisor, a drug dealer higher up the chain who had come in after hearing the commotion and proceeded to lambast the errant watcher. "No way are we calling 911," the guy said.

I interject to say that calling 911 for an overdose comes with immunity from prosecution. My passenger shakes his head: "This is a drug house."

"Point taken," I say.

He goes on to describe the argument they had and how, in the end, the staff took the overdose victims outside and laid them in the snow. This is, of course, the same street where I had the encounter with the man who had lost his false teeth.

My partner and I drive down Hungerford Street later that day. I keep my eye out for bags. Sure enough I find a yellow bag with "The Finals" stamped on it. The Finals is a logo referring to the NBA tournament. The next day I find Star Wars. My collection is up to date again, and the mystery of the guy with the false teeth seems to be explained.

My theory is that they gave both patients Narcan. The guy with the false teeth was left in the snow on the same street, probably because he was coming around. The second guy perhaps was carried or driven farther away, as he was still not breathing. Whether he died in the house or later out in the snow, I don't know. It seems likely that his death could have been prevented if someone competent in the drug house had been watching over him and had immediately given him Narcan or had called 911 for help.

I am at the pavilion next to the pond at Pope Park looking for needles and any bags of new brands of heroin when I see two young men hurrying across the park toward me. "What's up?" I ask.

"Hey, what's up?" one of the men says back.

"Nothing, just enjoying the day. You staying safe?"

"Yeah, we're glad to have you around. You're like our security guard." The second young man looks a little concerned to see a tall person in uniform, but the other guy reassures him: "He's cool; no worries, man."

Without another word, they both get down on the cement, one sitting and the other kneeling, and they take out a syringe and a bottle-cap-sized cooker. I watch as one man rips open two bags of heroin and drops their contents into the cooker and squirts in some saline from a blue vial. I am fascinated by what I am witnessing but am uncertain about the ethics of my standing in uniform next to two people using illegal drugs. I say, "Be safe. I'll be up in the ambulance. Call me if you need me."

"Go on and do it already," the first young man says. He has already tied a USB cord around his arm and is holding his arm out for his friend to inject him.

I sit in the ambulance and watch them from fifty yards away. One's head drops forward while the other stands, stretches, and looks off across the pond at birds flying out of the marsh grass, perhaps after being startled by a predator. A few minutes later he helps his buddy up, and they throw their backpacks over their shoulders and march back across the field. No overdose this time. The scene will become commonplace.

When I walk through the park to stretch my legs, my radio hanging on my belt, I walk past users nodded out on benches. Some have their own chaperones, men I recognize from Park Street, who lean against a vacant building or in the window of a car. I am guessing this is an enhanced service. Buy some dope from the dealer, and he or one of his boys will sit with you to make certain you don't OD or get robbed if you nod out. Sometimes, if users are nodded out alone, I ask them if they are all right. They open their eyes, mumble, and go back to their bliss. Every now and again, I have to give one a gentle shake. "Just checking to see if you are okay. No worries here," I say. Sometimes in winter, if it is bitterly cold, I will lay a blanket on one.

Statistics for 2016 from the state Office of Emergency Medical Services show that 62 percent of overdoses in the state of

Connecticut occur in people's homes, while in the city of Hartford, 53 percent of overdoses take place in public.[1] More recent data from the Hartford Opioid Project show that nearly 70 percent of all opioid overdoses in Hartford occur outside the overdosed person's home.[2] The Hartford figures are higher than those for the state because of the many homeless people who are addicted to heroin and because so many people come into Hartford from the suburbs to buy heroin. When they are in a state of withdrawal, many use the drug before leaving the city. They may then overdose in a fast-food restaurant bathroom, at a bus stop, or in their car. The amount of heroin consumed within the city limits results in so many heroin bags littering the ground that my partners and I amend the rules for our heroin bag hunt: now you get bonus points if you step on a heroin bag when you get out of the ambulance. One day I even find a heroin bag up on the Interstate 91 overpass when we are on the scene of a car accident.

One of the most popular injection sites in Hartford is a portable toilet. I drink fluid (tea, water, sometimes Diet Coke) all day long. I try to pee when I am at the hospital, but sometimes I have to go when I am away from the hospital. I use a portable toilet in a park when I really need to go. The problem is that I have to compete with heroin users for the toilets. On more times than I can count, I have opened the door of a portable toilet with a broken lock to find someone inside injecting. Now I always knock. Often I hear a panicked "Occupied!" After walking back to the ambulance, I have watched users come out of the toilet and make their way off to wherever it is they dig up their next four dollars. The portable toilets are rich hunting grounds for the latest heroin bags, as users often crumple up their empty bags and toss them in the urinal or on the floor. They also leave their syringes.

I am training a new medic, Daniel Hammersmith. I teach him about stroke and cardiac care, about handling a multi-vehicle car accident, and also about the opioid epidemic and heroin bags. We are in Bushnell Park, our ambulance in the shade by the Soldiers and Sailors Memorial Arch. Dan says he is going to take a walk over to the portable toilets. There was a big event that weekend in the park, and there is a line of ten toilets where there are normally only two. "Bring back a new heroin bag," I say.

When Dan reaches the portable toilets, he notices that the door of one is not fully closed. A sneaker blocks it. He opens the door, and an unresponsive man tumbles out. A syringe and empty heroin bags lie on the floor. The man is blue and breathes only with stimulation. One shake, one breath. Dan radios us that he has an OD. Bryan drives the ambulance over the sidewalk to get closer. I get out the house bag and bring it over to where Dan is vigorously shaking the man to keep him breathing. I get out an Ambu bag and start breathing for the patient, while Dan takes out the naloxone.

Just then, I notice another man sprinting frantically across the park directly toward us. The running man stops and stands a few feet away, looking hard at the overdose victim, whose face is covered by a mask. I lift the mask briefly to let the man look. "You know this guy?" I ask.

"No," he shakes his head. "I thought it was Doug." A moment later, the door of another portable toilet opens, and a man stumbles out. He looks dazed.

"Doug!" the other man shouts. "You're all right. I thought this dude was you."

Doug looks at us bagging the patient. "Fuck," he says.

With naloxone in his system, our patient starts breathing better on his own. His level of carbon dioxide has dropped from 100 to 48. He is now ventilating himself adequately. We lift our patient up on the stretcher and wheel him toward the ambulance.

During the commotion a large flatbed truck has backed down the sidewalk. The crane on the back lifts a portable toilet from the row and places it on the back of the truck. Our patient opens his eyes now and looks about. "Oh, Christ!" he swears. "You guys Narcaned me, didn't you?"

"Believe it or not," Dan says, watching the last portable toilet raised into the air, "it's your lucky day." Another fifteen minutes and our patient would have been out of our zip code.

In Vancouver, Canada, there is a place called Insite, which is a government-run safe-injection site founded in 2003. It is located in the heart of the city's drug district. There, users can enter a clean building where they can get fresh needles, sterile water, cookers, alcohol wipes, and new tourniquets. There are twelve stalls where users can sit and inject. Afterward, they move to another room, where they can wait until they are ready to leave. At all times, they are under the watchful eyes of health workers who monitor them for overdose and who are there to counsel them if desired—teaching them safe-injection practices or offering to get them into detox or medication-assisted therapy such as Suboxone or methadone.[3] Since Insite started, there have been over 6,440 overdoses on the premises. Not a single person has died.[4]

The safe-injection site is on the first floor. On the second floor of the same building is Onsite, a twelve-bed detox center. On the third floor is transitional recovery housing, where patients are assisted with getting into longer-term programs, housing, and support.[5]

A study published in *The Lancet* in 2016 compared the overdose rate in Vancouver's drug district in the two years before the opening of Insite with the rate in the two years after Insite opened and found that it had decreased by 35 percent.[6] Other studies showed that the supervised injection site had led to a greater chance of users getting off drugs and to increased use of treatment services.[7,8]

A study in the *Harm Reduction Journal* did a cost-benefit analysis of how much a similar safe-injection site would benefit the city of Baltimore, Maryland, which has one of the worst overdose death date rates in the country. The study looked at six different benefits: preventing the spread of the human immunodeficiency virus, hepatitis C, skin and soft-tissue infections, and overdose deaths; decreasing costs associated with nonfatal overdoses; and enabling people to get into medication-assisted therapy. The study found that for an investment of $1.8 million, a safe-injection site would save $7.8 million in costs, prevent deaths, reduce infections, limit days spent in a hospital for skin infections, reduce ambulance runs, decrease emergency room (ER) use and hospital admission, and get more people into treatment.[9]

In Hartford, there is a four-story community health center on Grand Street, a road that runs parallel to Park Street one block to the north. Next to the health center is an abandoned building with trees and overgrown weeds in its back lot. From the higher floors on the east side of the center, staff can observe users walking through the weeds to the back porch or squatting under the trees, where they shoot up. One afternoon a staff member calls in an OD after observing a patient lying still under a tree after having a seizure. We respond and revive the patient with naloxone. On the way to the hospital, he mentions that the heroin bag he used was branded "Satan." Since it is a brand I don't know, my partner and I go back to the site after we clear the hospital. We find five users in various states of injecting. One man is drawing back a syringe's plunger, and we can see blood in the chamber as he checks to see whether he's got the needle securely in a vein. Another man shudders after injecting and then is still, other than the slow movement of his chest. It is a baking-hot day, and they all seem too tired to flee from our presence. "It's okay," I say. "Peace be with you all." We go back to the truck, and since it is nearly 90 degrees, I have a cooler of water bottles packed in ice, which we bring back around to the circle of users. I am a poor man's philanthropist. I get as much satisfaction in giving a water bottle beaded with condensation to a thirsty person as I expect Bill Gates might get from giving someone a six-figure check. People don't expect cold water to materialize in their hand on a sizzling day. We pass out the cold bottles to the users, which they are thrilled with. They help me find a Satan bag and agree to be careful should they encounter it. I wish I could leave them naloxone, but two of the five show me their Narcan kit.

The next day we are up on the third floor of the health center to pick up a hypertensive patient from one of the treatment rooms, and we can look out the window and see the users gathered in the back lot. The staff tell us that they called in an overdose yesterday. We reply that we were the ones who responded and that the patient did well. "It's terrible," the nurse says, "what goes on there."

"Do you know what you could do to help?" I say. "You could open up one of the first-floor exam rooms and let them shoot up in the health center instead of in the weeds. You could give them clean needles, tourniquets, and alcohol wipes. You can treat their abscesses and have a social worker help them find housing. You can offer to get them into rehab. And if they overdose, you can revive them with naloxone. One-stop shopping. You can treat them like you treat all your patients here, with kindness and without judgment."

She looks at me like I have three heads. "Ha ha," she says. "I don't think so."

"But really," I say, "don't you think that would be a great idea? You could help people and save lives."

"Heroin is illegal," she says sternly. "That'll never fly."

"A shame," I say, "but a man can dream."

It has been reported that many cities in America have discussed opening their own safe-injection sites, but no one wants to be the first.[10] The problems are twofold. One is political. Many citizens don't want one in their neighborhood. They might change their mind, though, if they learned that, after some initial trepidation, the neighborhood in Vancouver actually embraced its safe-injection site. They decided that it is better to have users shooting up inside the building than behind a trash can in an alley. The second, and more powerful, problem is legal. There is a fear that the operators of a safe-injection site could be arrested and charged with running a drug house under section 856 of the federal drug statute, known colloquially as the crack house statute.[11] US deputy attorney general Rod Rosenstein tells National Public Radio, "I'm not aware of any valid basis for the argument that you can engage in criminal activity as long as you do it in the presence of someone with a medical license." He warns states considering legalizing such sites to consult their state attorney general about legal repercussions, including criminal prosecution that could come from Washington.[12]

In October 2019, a federal judge rules that Safehouse, a non-profit group in Philadelphia, is not violating the law with its proposed safe-injection site in a neighborhood plagued by overdose deaths. The crack house statute prohibits the operation of a space "for the purpose of manufacturing, distributing or using controlled substances." US district judge Gerald McHugh writes, "The ultimate goal of Safehouse's proposed operation is to reduce drug use, not facilitate it."[13]

The federal government vows to appeal this ruling, and the Office of the Attorney General threatens to shut down any attempt to open such a site. US deputy attorney general Jeffrey Rosen declares, "Any attempt to open illicit drug injection sites in other jurisdictions while this case is pending will continue to be met with immediate action by the department." The threat of Washington hurling a thunderbolt at an effort to help America's most vulnerable citizens is unnerving for many in harm reduction. It is hard to stand up to people who have the power to crush you.

A recent study suggests that people would be more willing to accept such a facility if it were simply to go by a different name.

When called an overdose prevention site, 45 percent of survey responders supported it, as opposed to only 21 percent when it was called a safe-injection site.[14]

The obstacles haven't deterred a number of people in the harm reduction community from opening up unofficial safe-injection sites. A study of one such facility appeared in the *American Journal of Public Health* in 2017.[15] The small unsanctioned site in an undisclosed American city has a room with five stations, where users can sit and, in clean surroundings, use sterile supplies provided by the site to inject drugs they have purchased outside the facility. A staff person trained in naloxone administration and rescue breathing, as well as harm reduction principles and safe-injection techniques, observes them. Eighty percent of the users are homeless, and in regular surveys nearly all report they would otherwise be injecting in public bathrooms, behind buildings, or in parks. Here they can take their time injecting and not be rushed. Rushing, of course, can lead to tissue damage when a user pushes a shot in without having the needle's point inside a vein. After visitors inject, the used syringes are safely discarded in a sharps box, not discarded in public as they otherwise might be.

Mark Jenkins is also an advocate for having a sanctioned safe-injection site in Hartford, but there are obstacles, just as there once were obstacles to running a needle exchange and to making naloxone available. Back then, early harm reductionists went ahead and did the exchanges and passed out naloxone on their own in acts of civil disobedience because they recognized their deeds were saving lives. What the hell else could they do?

In 2016, the US government ended its ban on federal funding for operating needle exchange programs, which were thriving despite a lack of federal funds.[16] The government still prevents federal funds from being spent on the syringes. Today, more than two hundred needle exchange programs operate in forty states.[17] The cost has been estimated to be $20 per user per year. The cost of treating one AIDS patient has been estimated at $120,000 a year.[18] Plus, research has shown that those who have used a needle exchange program are five times more likely to get into treatment than those who haven't.[19] Needle exchange programs provide a community and a sense of caring. By seeing users on a regular basis, workers build trust and a friendship with them; users come to see the workers as a helping hand, available should they decide they want help for their addiction. Once needle exchange programs, like naloxone distribution, were illegal. Today they are saving lives. Safe-injection sites are the next logical step and a proven commonsense approach in the fight to save lives.

I write an op-ed that gets published in the *Hartford Courant* titled "I See What Heroin Does: Let People Shoot Up Safely." In it, I argue that Hartford should "designate a safe house where heroin users can inject while monitored by a health professional for accidental overdose." I describe overdosed patients I have treated behind abandoned buildings and in park bushes, discuss how addiction is a disease and not a character flaw, cite the number of deaths in Connecticut, and mention the danger to the public of heroin bags, syringes, and other drug debris. I conclude, "A safe injection site won't drop the death rate to zero, but we can save some lives and get this hard-to-reach population into treatment. That's no small achievement."[20] An accompanying sidebar, "5 Things to Know about Opioid Addiction," shows photos of a number of the heroin bags I have collected.[21]

Yet, for all the talk, no official, legal safe-injection site has opened in the United States. New York, Philadelphia, and Seattle all have announced their intentions to open sites, but all the efforts have stalled in bureaucracy, red tape, and for fear of federal retaliation.

I spend a day on the needle exchange van at Park and Hungerford with two harm reduction workers, Norm Lebron and LaToya Tyson. Users turn in their needles and get clean ones along with antibiotics, sterile cookers, and some gentle conversation about how they are doing.

"You guys are great!" a jittery young man says. "I used to come down here and shoot up all the time. You got me straight. I've been doing good, real good, getting my life back together. I'm only here today to get needles for my brother. Not for me. I'm working on getting him clean. I don't want him down here. He comes down here, he may never come back. It's rough on these streets. I was homeless down here. I don't want him getting sucked in." He empties twenty syringes from his backpack and is given two ten-packs of sterile syringes along with tourniquets and a couple of cookers. As the exchange is made, I look at the crook of his elbow and see fresh needle marks.

LaToya and Norm tell me about others they have seen who have made it—those who are no longer using and who are working and have families. These people have expressed their gratitude for having help through a difficult period of their lives. And even those who continue to use are grateful that there are people out there who care about them, who recognize their humanity, and who know that every day spent alive on earth is something to be thankful for.

I watch as the users disperse. Some go into alleys to shoot up behind a dumpster; others go into a public restroom or down into the underbrush off Park Terrace to sit on an old tire or milk crate and inject in the company of flies circling deposits of feces. There is a disconnect here: we give them sterile equipment to ward off disease and keep them alive, but then we cast them out to shoot up in the most unsterile of places.

I try to stop by the van on days I am working on the ambulance. Mike Grace and Sue Levin are on the van on Tuesdays. Like Norm and LaToya, they are true front-line workers in this great epidemic. I understand their frustration about inaction and talk. They see the users every day, see how they deteriorate, while too few are steered to rehab. They hear of deaths of some who overdosed alone and died because no one found them in time.

On Albany Avenue, Mark Jenkins opens up a walk-in center. People can get coffee and sit down out of the sun or cold. There is a counselor on hand to help people get into rehab if they are tired of the life they are living. I stop by occasionally. The place is always crowded, and people seem happy there. It is a safe place. There are clean needles and other supplies. A shower is available for the homeless and a bathroom.

When we talk about safe-injection sites, Mark says there are consumption places all over the city—parks, alleys, public restrooms, and cars—but they are not safe places. Alex Diaz sits outside Mark's bathroom. What goes on in his bathroom may be no different from what goes on in the restroom of the Subway restaurant down the street, in the McDonald's on Washington Street where several people have lost their lives, or in the restrooms of the public library on Main Street, which is a site from which 911 overdose calls are frequent. The only difference is a man who sits outside the bathroom and counts the time. If you are in there past three minutes, he knocks on the door and says, "Friend, are you all right?"

Cut

Here is a partial list of ingredients that heroin has been known to be cut with:

acetaminophen, aspirin, baby formula, baking powder, Benadryl, caffeine, cocaine, corn starch, dextromethorphan (cough suppressant), ephedrine, flour, gabapentin (anti-epileptic), kratom (psychotropic plant), laundry detergent, levamisole (medicine for parasitic worm infections), laxative, mannitol (artificial sweetener), methamphetamine, powdered milk, quinine, strychnine (rat poison), sugar, talc, Xylocaine (numbing agent)

There are several reasons why dealers cut their heroin with other ingredients. One reason is to increase the bulk. If you have 100 grams of heroin and you add an equal amount of cut, you then have 200 grams. A $5 bag of heroin usually contains 0.1 gram of powder. Once the cut is added, a thousand bags of heroin become two thousand bags of heroin with additive. The problem is this: the more cut you add, the more you decrease the strength of the heroin; pretty soon, your product is so weak that no one will want to buy it, particularly if others are selling stronger heroin. The general strength of the heroin on the local market tends to keep dealers from cutting too much if they want to move product.

Dealers do have an alternative to inactive cut. They can add active ingredients to strengthen or give zest to their product. Benadryl, for instance, adds a pleasing rush. And dealers have long added fentanyl to their batches of heroin. This practice led in many areas to fentanyl almost replacing heroin. Lately, in Hartford, dealers have been adding some weird unknown substance to heroin that is turning users into zombies.

A call takes us to a small park on Hudson Street, where a woman lies on the ground with agonal breathing. We revive her with naloxone and put her in the back of the ambulance. She looks at me as if I'm a creature from outer space. She does not speak, even though her eyes are open and her breathing returns to normal. I try to talk calmly to her, but she looks terrified. At the hospital, I tell the triage nurse that she may be on something else or suffering from some kind of trauma. We got a report that there were three men with her who fled when the fire department arrived before us. The next day, we are parked across from Pope Park in a little dirt turnaround. Bryan and I like to park here, stand outside the ambulance, and watch the people walk past. We often carry fruit or cold water to hand out. We try to make eye contact with users, some of whom stop and chat as we hand them something to eat or drink. I see a familiar-looking woman coming down the street, and she looks like she is coming over to talk. "I want to thank you," she says. "Thank you for helping me." She introduces herself as Gloria.

"I'm glad you're doing better," I say.

"I couldn't talk to you yesterday. They put something in the heroin. I think it was PCP, but I felt trapped in my body. I could see you, but I couldn't talk." I tell her that we have had other patients who have acted oddly of late. They are revived with naloxone but are almost catatonic. "It's a mind fuck," she tells us, "whatever they are putting in there. I don't like it."

The next week, as we are driving by the pavilion, I see what looks like a woman lying on the ground and a large man standing over her. I have Bryan circle back around. We park at the curb and both walk over with our portable radios in hand. It's Gloria. She has that same trapped-in-her-body look. The man lingers on the periphery. We help her up and walk her back up to the road. I offer to take her to the hospital, but she shakes her head and then moves off up the street. We both find it very odd.

The next day she stops by and is completely normal. She thanks us again and tells us that she had some more of the bad dope. She tells us that the dealer told her today there were both PCP (a hallucinogen) and THC (the psychoactive compound in marijuana) in the mix. She had asked for a different brand and says she should have known it was the same bad dope when he smiled at her. She tells us that she thought the man at the pavilion was going to rape her because she was trapped in her body.

Gloria becomes one of our regulars. We usually see her in the morning. She is a sex worker. She says that she makes up to three hundred dollars a night, but by morning she is usually close to broke because she uses most of her profits to buy drugs. She tells us she became addicted after having surgery when she was young. She met a man in rehab, and they got clean together. She was a housewife in the suburbs, and he worked in construction. They had a child together. Then the previous winter, when driving home from a Christmas party, her husband got pulled over for having a burned-out taillight. The police officer smelled alcohol on him and made him take a breathalyzer test. He blew over the limit. After having his name searched in the law enforcement database, the officer learned that he was in the country illegally. When he came to the United States from Brazil twenty years before as a boy with his family, the paperwork wasn't filled out right. Her husband was deported, and Gloria's life quickly fell apart. She's been on the streets for five months now. Her son lives with her sister, who won't let her see him. I imagine her as a housewife, hanging up clothes on the line, taking their ten-year-old son to his soccer games, hosting a dinner party, having a drink too many and getting giggly with her friends, vowing to start taking an aerobics class. She is about 20 pounds overweight now, she says, but promises me she was much curvier in her prime. She says she was proud of what she looked like.

I wonder what she will look like a year or two from now. Having tracked users over time, I know how rapidly they age. Their faces become lined; their eyes recede. Those who are homeless are sunburned and weather beaten, while those with homes become ghostly pale. You see the abscesses on their arms; some walk with a limp if they have started to inject in the veins of their legs. I think of the Richard Gere and Julia Roberts movie *Pretty Woman*, the modern-day *My Fair Lady*, when I look at Gloria or my friend Chloe, who is also a sex worker. In that movie, Richard Gere transforms Julia from a wisecracking, gum-smacking streetwalker dressed in stereotypical hooker attire into a wisecracking, champagne-sipping beauty in a thousand-dollar designer dress. Would it be possible to do the same for a user? If you were a person of unlimited resources, could you take a user off the street, clean her up, give her good medical care, house her, and get her a job with an understanding employer? If you could do all this, could you return her to what she once was or allow her to develop how she would have if drugs had not derailed her life? Or has the damage already been done, her brain irreparably rewired by opioids? In a remake of *Pretty Woman* truer to life, Richard Gere would come home from his day at the investment firm, and instead of finding a gorgeous Julia Roberts—waiting for him seductively, wearing only one of his dress shirts and a necktie—he would instead find her overdosed in the bathroom, face pressed against the ceramic toilet seat, blue, with vomit matting her hair. Would that be the end of the courtship for Gere, or would he not give up hope?

I wonder how Julia Roberts's character would handle an episode that Chloe tells me happened to her.

Chloe is picked up by two guys who immediately pull the car onto the highway and take her down to Bridgeport, a Connecticut city similar to Hartford, an hour to the south. There they hold her in a house for two days before finally returning her dope sick to Hartford without any payment for her services or time. When I tell her she needs to find new work, she admits that things have been hard for her lately. Business is slow. "I've lost a lot of weight. I've got no boobs anymore, and I have these scabs all over my face," she says. If Richard Gere's character wanted to save Chloe or Gloria, he'd need time, patience, and an abiding faith in human kinship, qualities more suited to a harm reductionist than a fictional financier. Recovery for users is never easy. Still, I think we should never quit on people or give anyone up for lost. They still need our best efforts, our love, even if the ending is not a happy one. I look forward to seeing Gloria on the days I work. "Stay away from that mind-fuck batch," I tell her.

"No worries. I won't ever buy from him again."

One morning, as we are on our way to a low-priority call, I see her stumble out of a car that speeds away. She crosses the street without looking and heads into the alley behind the Bean Pot Restaurant. She needs her fix and is at the mercy of whatever ingredients are in that small $4 envelope.

Harm reductionists have suggested that public health departments or community harm reduction organizations buy gas chromatography machines. The machine could be placed in a walk-in center in a high-use neighborhood so that street drugs could be tested to determine their ingredients. Such devices would not only detect impurities and novel adulterants but could also detect the presence of carfentanil. This information could then be spread to help keep people alive. From the state that has been the hardest hit by carfentanil deaths, Dennis Cauchon, the president of Harm Reduction Ohio, recently wrote, "Public health officials should consider allowing—indeed, encouraging—drugs to be tested for safety on the many gas chromatography–mass spectrometry machines that exist. Testing drugs for safety is now criminalized, a deadly health policy mistake. In reality, a gas chromatography machine costs just $20,000 or so and can do the job with great accuracy."[1] If dealers knew that what they are selling is being tested, they might stop putting crap into their product.

Mickey is walking down a side street off Park when he freezes in place. He sees a slow-moving black Toyota blink its lights, and then he sees a station wagon. Before he can take a step to flee, he sees a gun barrel poke out of the back window. He feels the impact against his shin and another in the hip. He dives behind the bus stop shelter as more bullets splat against the wall of the boarded-up store behind him. He scrambles up and runs into the street. He takes the orange he has in his pocket and heaves it at the car. Then he holds up double-barreled middle fingers. "Fuck you!" he shouts. "Your product sucks!"

"Five times I've been ambushed this week," he explains to me that afternoon. "He hit me eight times. Hurts like a mother. Look at me; I'm covered in paint. He uses a different car for his shooters every time. He flickers his lights to give them the signal, the bastard."

Mickey is a homeless addict who is a fixture on Park Street. He is short, wiry, and missing most of his teeth. Every six months he disappears for a while, going to stay with his aunt in a rural town in the northeastern part of the state. Invariably, I see him back on Park Street. He doesn't want to be an addict for the rest of his life, but staying with his aunt in the country makes him stir-crazy. He has nowhere to go in the town. He can't drive, he has no friends, and there are only so many chores you can do and so much TV you can watch. He gets the urge to call old friends, and then he messes up and is back on Park Street. Park Street has heroin, and he knows heroin will kill him one day. (He's already had a heart valve replaced because of endocarditis.) But on Park Street, Mickey is somebody. He has acquaintances. People know his name, even if one of them is trying to hit him with paintballs.

The attacks started a week ago. A few days before that, when he couldn't find his normal dealer, Mickey bought a bag from another dealer he knew. "Four dollars," the guy told him. "It's great. Four dollars. It's not cut with that crazy stuff. You'll love it." Mickey forked over his bills. The batch gave him what he called a "bad weed high." He felt all dark and paranoid, almost catatonic, all the while his heart was racing. He felt like crap for the rest of the day. When he tried to get his $4 back, the dealer told him to fuck off, so Mickey spent the better part of two days telling everyone on the street that this dealer's product sucked. Now, no one will buy it. The dealer even changed his brand's name and still has no takers. Mickey has a big mouth. He laughs when he tells the story. "So he's pissed at me."

"You have to be careful you don't get hit in the face."

"All the shots so far have been below the waist. That's the code. I'm worried he's going to get me in the nuts. I got newspaper there for padding."

I laugh over the comic manner of Mickey's storytelling and the thought of a pissed-off drug dealer chasing down a wise-guy half-pint with a paintball gun. Mickey's a tough guy, and he uses humor as a shield against the cold realities of his life. Despite his bravado, I have also seen him cry when talking about all the times he's been beaten up for fun, and I've seen him sick and looking like death as he waited desperately to find an open bed in Connecticut's overtaxed recovery system.

I hope the feud ends quickly and that Mickey's tormentor forgives him. As painful as paintballs can be, I am glad they are not bullets. Mickey at least knows there are few dealers he can trust and the ingredients of a bag of heroin will always be a surprise.

Danger Ahead

We arrive after the police and fire departments. A bearded boy, who looks familiar to me, sits against the door in the hallway crying and looking scared. A police officer stands over him. "Is this the OD?" I ask.

The officer shakes his head and nods into the apartment. On the living room floor another young man lies on his back, his arms outstretched. He is very pale. A firefighter stands over him trying to assemble an Ambu bag while another firefighter attaches a hose to the oxygen tank in his blue house bag. I see a discarded vial of Narcan by the young man's head. I look at him carefully. He looks dead. "Is he breathing?" Just then, I see his Adam's apple move with one agonal breath. The firefighters start bagging him. I attach the carbon dioxide monitor. It reads 100. "Any paraphernalia?" I ask.

"They all deny drug use." I see a girl crying on the couch.

"What did he use?" I ask her.

"I don't know. I just had a beer. He just fell over, and his friend told me to call 911." His blood pressure is good; his heart is going at 112. His pupils are pinpoint.

I go out into the hall and ask the boy, "What did he use?"

"I can't answer that."

"We're just trying to help him."

"I, I think I need to consult with my lawyer," he says.

"You're not in trouble. He's not under arrest, is he?" The officer shakes his head. The boy avoids my eyes. He looks familiar to me.

"Is your name Bart?" I ask. He looks down and doesn't answer. The cop reads his license.

"Bartholomew Johnston," he announces.

"I thought I recognized you," I say. "Call your parents when you get to the hospital and tell them you're okay."

I go back in the room and see the young man's carbon dioxide is down to 50. I give him a sternal rub, but he doesn't respond. The carbon dioxide drops to around 40. I tell them to stop bagging. His respiratory rate is now 16. His oxygen saturation is 100; carbon dioxide, 42. He is stable.

I go back outside. "Your friend is fine. He responded to Narcan. What did the bag look like that you bought?"

"You can tell us," the cop says. "You're not under arrest. It's just to help your friend." Bart looks uncertain.

"You are going to be in trouble if you don't help," the cop says.

"It was a clear bag," he says. "We just bought cocaine. He wanted to do some. It was his idea."

"Cocaine, huh," I say. "Seems there was probably some fentanyl in it."

"There was no fentanyl in it," Bart says.

"How do you know that?" the cop asks.

"I used to do pills and heroin," he says.

"Does your friend do it, too?"

"No, just cocaine, and he smokes pot."

"Well, something got in the mix. Be careful what you buy these days."

The friend finally arouses, but he is too groggy to walk. We stair-chair him down the three flights and take him to the hospital.

"What happened," the boy says, once in the ambulance. "Was I in a car accident?"

"You overdosed on an opioid," I say.

"What?"

This isn't the first time that people in Hartford have bought what they thought was cocaine but ended up having either heroin with fentanyl or cocaine laced with heroin and fentanyl. It is almost impossible to tell white heroin, fentanyl, and cocaine apart by sight.

What happened to the boys? Did the dealer think Bart said *dope* instead of *coke*? Did he sell him coke that he had spiked with fentanyl? Did someone higher up the chain do it? Or was it contaminated at the drug-packaging site? Did they neglect to clean the grinder and the scale they used for fentanyl before they started packaging their cocaine, resulting in cross-contamination?

There has been a lot of speculation about this issue. Mark Jenkins thinks it is accidental contamination. He says it doesn't make sense that a dealer would add fentanyl to cocaine, which might kill a customer who is opioid naive. In this case he is right: when lab test results come back for the two patients, Bart tests positive only for cocaine, while his friend tests positive for both cocaine and fentanyl.

Whether deliberate or unintentional, these overdoses are increasing. Not just in Hartford but across the country. Anyone buying or using cocaine these days needs to be careful.

A high school senior is found passed out in his bedroom with agonal breathing. "He doesn't use heroin!" his mother screams. "I know. I use. He doesn't. He just likes benzos. Narcan won't work."

"Is there a chance he got into your stash?" I ask as I hit him with 1.2 milligrams of naloxone in the thigh.

"No, I don't have a stash."

"His friends just dropped him off. None of them uses heroin. It's pills."

"He was out all night?"

"He's eighteen," she says. "I can't keep track of him. I'm not responsible for his actions."

This is a house where we have revived others before, including his mother. "I'm not judging," I say. "I'm just trying to get information."

We breathe for him, and in a matter of minutes, his respirations pick back up. Then suddenly he becomes combative, and it takes three firefighters and my partner to hold him down. A police officer holds the mother back to keep her from interfering with us. The young man finally stops fighting and then lies there panting.

"Did you use heroin?" I ask.

"I don't do heroin," he says. "Leave me the fuck alone. I'm in my own house."

"You're going to the hospital," the police officer says, and "you're not giving anyone a hard time." He says it with such authority that the young man complies. I sense that the officer and he have a history.

"Tell the medic what you used," the officer says.

"Xanax. I bought a couple bars off a guy I met at the party I was at."

"You must have done an opioid because you weren't breathing and naloxone revived you."

"No, I told you, only Xanax and a couple beers."

"Don't lie to us."

"No," I say, holding my hand up. "He could be telling the truth."

At a recent conference I attended, Robert Lawlor, a special agent with an organization called the New England High Intensity Drug Trafficking Area, told us about fentanyl being put in pills and sold as counterfeit drugs: oxycodone, Percocet, Xanax. The pills, he said, were remarkably similar to the real thing. Some might look like the pill had been in someone's pocket for a few days. He even showed us pictures of a pill press his organization had helped to impound and a vat full of counterfeit pills. This, he said, was the new wave.

The economics behind it are stunning. You can buy an industrial pill press along with some pill dies on the internet for a couple thousand dollars. A kilogram of pure fentanyl costs four thousand dollars. Add a couple hundred dollars for cutting agents like baby formula, and you are in business. According to the Drug Enforcement Administration, a kilogram of fentanyl broken down into a milligram per pill would yield one million counterfeit pills. At a street cost of twenty dollars per pill, an investment of several thousand dollars can generate up to twenty million dollars in profit.[1]

Just as fentanyl mixes poorly in powder, the same thing happens when fentanyl is pressed into pills. It's the chocolate chip scenario of uneven distribution. There is no quality control to ensure an even mix of ingredients. Instead of 1 milligram, you could get 2 milligrams in one pill—a lethal dose for some. An analysis by the Drug Enforcement Administration of twenty-six seized fentanyl-containing pills found an average of 1.1 milligrams per pill but a range from 0.03 to 1.99 milligrams.[2] Clumpy fentanyl makes each pill a death lottery. The Xanax bar or Percocet you buy from a street source could just be fentanyl plus cut, and it could be the last pill you ever take.[3] The rock legend Prince reportedly died from taking a Vicodin that he likely had no idea was counterfeit. It was a deadly dose of fentanyl.[4]

While I have not seen it in Hartford, a user I met who lives in Rhode Island tells me he has seen dealers use special dies to press pills containing methamphetamine into novelty shapes and colors like a yellow Sponge Bob pill and a pink Joker face in a new method of drug branding. I hate to think about a child finding one of these on the floor or in the grass at a park. They look like Flintstone vitamins.

The Bakery

In the Merrie Melodies cartoon "Sheep Ahoy," Ralph Wolf and Sam Sheepdog go to work each morning and exchange greetings while punching the clock.

"Morning, Ralph," the sheepdog says.

"Morning, Sam," the wolf replies.

Then it is down to business. The wolf spends his hours trying to steal the sheep, and the sheepdog spends his hours trying to stop the wolf. At the end of the day, after the factory whistle blows, Ralph and Sam punch out, wishing each other a good night, before presumably heading home to their families, a hot dinner, and a sound sleep. They will return the next day to do it all over again.

It is a vision of the world that I would like to believe in. I sometimes think of Hartford in the same terms. In the morning at the bakery on Park Street, there are drug dealers, drug users, police, and paramedics all in line for their coffee, doughnuts, or breakfast sandwiches. Everyone is convivial. Then it is off to work. The dealers try to sell their product, the cops try to stop them. The users try to use, and we try to see that no one gets hurt.

When I respond to city lockups or arrive on arrest scenes where we may have been called to evaluate a person in handcuffs who fell during a foot pursuit, there is often a common courtesy, even friendliness, among everyone, in the same way that players from rival sports teams may chat at halftime or during time-outs. This, of course, is not always true, as oftentimes rival teams engage in chest puffing and taunting. Still, I like to think there is a comradeship among us all who belong to the same city and same species. I remember when the University of Connecticut men's basketball team won its first national championship in 1999, shocking the country by upsetting Duke, everyone in the jailhouse was in high spirits, cops and robbers both saying, "How about those Huskies!"

An idealist, I believe that we are all, at essence, just people following the course of our lives, which we don't always control. The cop came from a family of cops; the drug dealer grew up in a family of drug dealers; and the drug user got too fond of the painkiller he was prescribed after an accident. I ended up in EMS because I watched the TV show *Emergency* and had a crush on nurse Dixie McCall, played by Julie London.

As a paramedic, I have treated many kinds of patients in my ambulance: injured cops, shot drug dealers, overdosed users, and fellow EMS responders with a blown-out back. They are all patients, and I treat them the same. We have conversations; we talk about our families. I believe there is a fundamental goodness in most of us. But clearly there is darkness in the world. There are cops who cross the line; there are paramedics who don't give a shit; and there are drug dealers without a conscience.

I take the position, however, that not all drug dealers are evil at core. Bear with me on this. Some dealers, I believe, are honest businesspeople who just want to make a living and who adhere to basic business ethics. They provide a product to people who would be sick without it, people who come to them freely. They pay their associates fairly; they charge fair market prices; and they deliver the product they advertise. They don't rip their customers off.

They develop a clientele, whom they look out for, sometimes extending credit during hard times, maybe giving them an extra bag at Christmas or on their birthday. These dealers do not want their customers to die. They want them to be happy, to feel passion, to find peace.

I ask Chloe if her drug dealers are ever kind. Some are, she says. "If I am really sick, and I didn't earn enough, they'll front me a bag, knowing I'm good for it. You can't take advantage of them, though. I may ask them to front me, maybe once a month. Some people who buy more from them, they'll front them more; it all depends on how much you buy. Other dealers, they sell you crap, even though they tell you it's good. They don't care; they just want your money; and they know you're desperate."

I ask Mark Jenkins for his perspective. He says that when a gang kid gets his stake from a larger dealer and the batch turns out to be bad, the kid is stuck with it and must recoup his money in some way. He needs to raise cash, and the only way he can do this is by selling his product, tainted or not. A more established street dealer can take the longer view. He knows that, in the end, he'll make more by being trustworthy. He can afford to take the hit of a bad batch. Over time, dealers and users can develop trust. Mark talks about setting up a system where dealers can bring their supply to harm reduction groups, who can have the batches tested with gas chromatography–mass spectrometry, and he is working with the state health department on just such a project. He is also working to see that drug dealers have access to naloxone and fentanyl test strips.

"It's all about keeping people alive," Mark says. "That is in everyone's interest."

Chris is a bearlike young man in his early twenties. But he has dropped close to 60 pounds in the year I have known him—a year of living on the streets, walking all over the city, and doing heroin.

He is nodded out at the bus stop on Main Street one day when I respond. I don't need to give him Narcan, just some stimulation to get his breathing back up to normal and bring him around. He doesn't want to go to the hospital, but we do have a long talk that day. He admits that he's been going hard at the heroin. "Even my dealer told me I needed to look at myself in the mirror and ask if I still wanted to live," he tells me. I give him the phone number of the opioid hotline and warn him never to do heroin alone.

Every time I see Chris after that, he thanks me for saving his life, when all I did was give him a couple of shakes and talk to him. Whenever I see him walking down Park Street, we pull up in the ambulance, and I ask him how he is doing. I know he appreciates that someone looks out for him, even if it is as simple as saying hello and asking how he's doing. He's been in and out of rehab twice in the time I've known him. When a few months pass and I haven't seen him, I think maybe he's dead or maybe his dealer talked him into going to rehab again. I like to think the latter. I like to think he has turned his life around.

Chris's dealer is a different breed from those who have only darkness in their hearts. Dark-hearted dealers are the ones spiking select bags of their heroin with extra fentanyl to cause fatal overdoses and increase word-of-mouth advertising for their brand.[1] Those predators are the ones who put carfentanil in their bags and stamp cartoon images of panda bears on them, which a child might find and think was powdered candy. They are the villains who cross the line in the same way that a rogue police officer delivers an unnecessary beat down or a paramedic lets a patient die out of laziness or spite. There was no pure evil in the world of Merrie Melodies, but that was just a cartoon, after all.

We receive a dispatch for an unresponsive overdose. We are coming from Newington, the next town over to the south. We are ten miles from the location, but we are the only unit available. I expect the dispatcher to radio us and ask for our estimated time of arrival or to update us on what is going on at the scene. There are no updates—no police department dispatcher asking if we are a medic unit or telling us Narcan was administered or that CPR is in progress. I am expecting the worst.

When we arrive, we see a fire engine and two police cars. People are gathered outside a triple-decker building, as word has no doubt gotten around the neighborhood. I know what we will find. A firefighter standing by the engine nods to us. A police officer comes out of the house and walks toward his cruiser. I grab my red house bag and cardiac monitor anyway and climb the narrow stairs and trudge down a hallway into an open boarding-house bedroom.

A man leans back against the bed like he had been sitting up and then just fell suddenly backward. He has rigor mortis and lividity. Asystole in all three leads. On his right shoulder is a giant New York Yankees tattoo. It's Berto. How awful. It is hard to picture this lifeless corpse as the smiling big man buying his pal, Lenny, a guava pastry at the bakery in the morning. That man has left. It is the tattoo that confirms the identity of a body whose soul has departed.

I announce the time. It doesn't take long to get a picture of what happened. On a small table is a cardboard box, the kind that glassine envelopes come in, and on top of the box is a small pile of white powder. A broken-off ballpoint-pen case used to snort the powder lies next to the box. In the trash can is a torn heroin bag with a faded red stamp I don't recognize. A firefighter tells me the patient overdosed a couple of days ago and was brought to the emergency department. In the corner of the room is a hospital gown with two electrodes still stuck to it. In a trash can, I see an Ambu bag and medical trash, including an open box of Narcan. A crew must have recently resuscitated him in this same room.

After I have given my info to the police for their report, which they will relay to the medical examiner, I walk back down the stairs. I see Lenny. He sits on the front steps, his head in his arms. I saw the two of them just a week ago at the bakery, getting coffee and the cheap bologna and cheese sandwiches that sell for $1.50. He looks up at me, but I cannot change what he already knows.

"I'm sorry," I say.

He nods. "He was supposed to meet me at a friend's house," Lenny says, "but he never showed."

"I'm sorry," I say again. I am tempted to sit down next to him and ask him about his and Berto's lives, but he looks back down at his hands. I leave him to his grief. I load my gear back into the ambulance, and we drive away, our lights off.

Tomorrow, a line will re-form at the bakery. People will punch the time clock. Users will use. Drug dealers will deal. Law enforcement will pursue. Paramedics will try to patch up the wounded. And, in Connecticut, three more people will die of overdose.

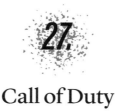

Call of Duty

A young man gets out of jail after spending thirty days inside for failing to appear in court on a traffic warrant. He gets picked up by acquaintances who, as a present, give him a $4 bag of heroin to snort. ("Just one bag," he tells me later, "and I snorted it. I've never OD'd before. And on top of that I've been clean for two months.")

His acquaintances are going to drop him off at his girlfriend's house. His girlfriend is going to drive him to his ex-wife's house. His ex-wife has agreed to let him take his eight-year-old son trick-or-treating. Instead, shortly after snorting the heroin, the man stops breathing and turns blue. His companions panic. They see a hospital sign up ahead. Unfortunately, it is no longer an emergency hospital; it serves primarily as a rehabilitation facility. They swerve into the hospital driveway, open the car door, and dump the man right in front of the main doors. They take off, leaving him face down on the pavement. A security guard comes out to investigate the sound of a car peeling away. He reaches the man prone on the ground and turns him over. The man is not breathing. The guard rushes back inside, alerts the medical staff, and calls 911.

Staff members come out pushing two crash carts. They get an Ambu bag out and start breathing for him. The fire department rolls in, and seeing the man apneic (his breathing arrested) and with pinpoint pupils, gives him 4 milligrams of Narcan up the nose.

When we arrive in the ambulance, I see a crowd gathered around the man. As I get to his side, he starts coming around. The firefighters stop bagging, and the man opens his eyes. I can see his panic. He is surrounded by medical personnel from the hospital and two crash carts. A nurse stands over him squeezing a bag of intravenous fluid. But that isn't what is scaring him. He is looking up at the Grim Reaper, a creepy-looking clown, and at least three ladies with a colorful cat face and whiskers. The facility is having a Halloween party.

"It's okay," I say to him. "You OD'd. They gave you Narcan. It's Halloween. You're all right now." I keep talking to him calmly as we get him on the stretcher and into the back of the ambulance. It takes a few minutes for him to realize what has happened.

"I'm a shit bag," he says to me. "I'm supposed to be taking my boy trick-or-treating tonight. I can't fucking believe I did this. You said I wasn't breathing. After all I've been through, to die like this. Fuck me. I've got shit for brains."

We talk on the way to the hospital. I ask the question I always ask: "How did you get started using opioids?"

"I broke my back when my Humvee hit an IED in an ambush," he says. "They think I might have gotten a brain injury. I had a bad concussion. They gave me butt loads of pain pills."

He was discharged with a purple heart and a bad painkiller habit. Veterans Administration staff tried to wean him off the painkillers, but they cut his amount too drastically. He had to buy pills on the street to keep from being dope sick. In no time, he was regularly driving into Hartford to buy heroin. His life quickly fell apart. He couldn't keep a job. His marriage ended. He slept on friends' couches until they kicked him out. He finally realized he would lose his son for good if he didn't get clean. He says he detoxed himself two months ago when he couldn't get into treatment. Withdrawal kicked his butt, but he fought through it. The cops stopped him for driving a car with a broken taillight, and his name came up as having an outstanding warrant. He had missed a court appearance for a traffic accident that happened when he nodded out behind the wheel after using. Getting out of jail today, when his buddies offered him a bag in celebration, he thought, What can one bag hurt?

When I put a cardiac electrode on his chest to the right of his sternum, the man flinches. He has a scar there. The scar is a bullet hole. "Twelve of us went over there together, but only three of us came back," he tells me. "And now I do this stupid shit."

At the ED, I give my report to Nancy and her trainee. Nancy rolls her eyes, but then I tell her the man's story. Whenever I turn an opioid user over to the hospital, I explain how the user got started so the nurse will better understand. I can see a change come over Nancy. Her husband is in the Army Reserves, and her brother served in Iraq. Once the man is placed in a room, my partner shakes the tearful man's hand and says, "Thank you for your service." So does the tech, Nancy, and her trainee.

It's only two o'clock in the afternoon. They'll observe him for a couple hours to make certain he doesn't go back out until the Narcan has worn off, and if he stays alert, they'll let him go. I know he wants to make it out in time to take his boy trick-or-treating. "You may make it yet," I say.

I tell his story when I speak before EMS groups. As a PowerPoint slide I have a picture of the Twin Towers in flames and Uncle Sam saying, "I want you." I address the group: "Tell me this man is a shit bag. He is a medical patient fighting a horrible brain disease of addiction that he contracted through no fault of his own. He gave our country his best. He, like every patient we ever touch, deserves ours."

A tall man in his early thirties, with a ghost-white complexion, stands on the side of the road, his head nodded forward, arms hanging down swaying. Another drug user on the nod in Hartford. I shake him. He opens his eyes and says he is fine, but then he drifts off again. My partner wheels the stretcher over, and we gently push him down onto it. He wakes again long enough to say he is fine, but he drops back out. In the ambulance, I check his respired carbon dioxide and his pulse saturation. The numbers are 66 and 90. When I stimulate him, the numbers come up a little, but if I leave him alone, he doesn't breathe well enough on his own. I put in an IV, which he doesn't feel. I take a 10 cc syringe, squirt out 1 cubic centimeter of saline solution, and then with a needle draw up 1 milligram of naloxone into the syringe. I slowly give him 1 cubic centimeter of the mixture, delivering 0.1 milligram of naloxone, a tiny dose. When he doesn't respond, I give him another 0.1 milligram, and soon he is talking to me. He doesn't even know I have given naloxone to him.

"I don't need to go to the hospital," he says. "What time is it? I have to get back to work or else I'm going to lose my job. I'm on my lunch break." It is three thirty in the afternoon. I ask him where he works, and he says he is a house painter. He asks where we picked him up. After I tell him, he says he is painting a house a few blocks from there. I tell him the doctors will look at him at the hospital and, after watching him for an hour, will let him go.

"Dude, I can't wait that long," he says, "I'll lose my job." I feel for him, but we have to take him in.

His name is Keith, and he lives in an upscale suburb of Hartford. His home address is familiar to me. I responded to an overdose on that same street maybe a year before. I remember the mother sobbing at the sight of her son on the bathroom floor, even though we were easily able to revive him. I sensed she was at her breaking point. He had already been through rehab four times.

"You didn't give me Narcan, did you?" Keith asks.

"Yes, I did," I say. "Just a little, enough to keep you breathing without me having to shake you every minute."

"Fuck. I'm going to lose my job."

"You have to be careful if you are going to use," I say.

"I only did a half a bag. I just haven't used. I got out of a program last week."

"Your tolerance is down. If you are going to use no matter what, have someone there with you. Have Narcan around. Do you have it at home?"

He nods.

"Who do you live with?"

"My dad took me back in."

"Does he know how to use it?"

"Yeah."

"You have to be careful with the fentanyl around."

"I know. My friend Marty died a month ago."

The name rings a bell with me. "What was his name?"

"Marty Harris."

"I took care of him before," I say. "That was a year ago." Marty was the young man I remembered. The news of his death, even though I barely knew him, shocks and saddens me. Marty and Keith are the same age.

"He got out of jail. After nine months, he OD'd and died."

"I'm sorry."

"Man, I'm going to lose my job."

Once we get to the hospital, he gets even more anxious, and he ends up pulling his IV out. I try to get a nurse to come over. I give the heads-up that he wants to leave. The nurse says he'll get a doctor to look at him. The doctor comes over, and the doctor and

Keith end up in a shouting match. The doctor tells Keith he obviously doesn't care about his own life because he is doing drugs that may kill him. The young man tells the doctor to fuck off and walks out, swearing that he is going to lose his job and now he has to walk all the way back to the job site.

That night I google his friend Marty's name and add the word *obituary* and the name of the town to the search terms. And there he is—a picture of the other young man. There is nothing in the obituary that mentions drugs. It just says he died too soon and what a kind heart he had. He was a high school swimmer, an avid soccer fan, and an accomplished cook. He liked to camp with his family in the Adirondacks. There is a long list of family members he left behind. I read the comments. One commenter says he remembers him fondly as a little boy playing in the neighborhood. There are pictures of him when he must have been about five. One shows him with a boy of a similar age, and I wonder whether it is the man I transported today. Another person comments, "He is no longer in pain."

I attend a conference where a father, John Lally, shows a video of the Today I Matter project in honor of his son Timothy, who succumbed to an overdose just shy of his thirtieth birthday.[1] The video shows the poster project, which is a traveling memorial where posters of loved ones lost to drugs are displayed together in a public place. Each poster features a photograph of someone who lost his or her life to overdose, along with the name of the person's town and two personal descriptors. Timothy's poster shows him playing his guitar. It says Timothy, Ellington, Artist/Musician. Other posters memorialize a Sister/Sea Lover, Joyful/Friend, Athlete/Charismatic, Great Laugh/Hard Worker, Pianist/Athlete, Gentle/Kind, Hero/Brave, Fisherman/Family Man, Engineer/Jokester, Free Spirited/Artistic. In the video, the camera lingers on each poster for several seconds before moving on to the next one. The posters are staked out in a large rectangle in an open field. As the camera moves along, you can hear a relentless wind.

I am on a panel at a community forum. A man asks us if we think it is true that people are only paying attention to the opioid epidemic because it now affects white people in the suburbs, while, when it affected people of color in the inner city, nobody cared. A panelist tells the audience that the War on Drugs began in the 1970s as a way of attacking black and poor people. She also cites the drastic differences in average jail sentences for possessing crack cocaine, a form of cocaine more common among blacks than whites, versus jail sentences for possessing powder cocaine, the form of the drug generally favored by whites. The disparity is a terrible miscarriage of justice in a country that professes to treat all citizens the same.

The woman is right, and I can sense her bitterness at the changing narrative. For years, people in the cities died, and no one seemed to care about the "addicts" and "junkies" who threw their lives away with poor choices. (I can say that those who died included all races.) That the opioid epidemic has gained attention in the suburbs to the point that people are now talking about it, and using their political power to fight on behalf of their addicted sons and daughters instead of disowning them, is not a bad thing. For years the suburbs were silent as their children died. While the death rate in the suburbs seems to be improving, similar gains are not happening in Hartford. Nationwide, the epidemic is growing in the inner cities. Will we as a nation—suburb and city—continue to speak out on behalf of all sufferers?

I would like to think that this crisis will bring us all together so that we treat everyone the same. There are millions out there in the cold who need our help to find their way home. This country and our military have a saying: "We leave no one behind." In EMS, as in all medicine, we have an obligation to honor the Hippocratic Oath: "Into whatsoever houses I enter, I will enter to help the sick."[2] That commitment must apply to all.

I have treated overdose cases of all races. I have found people dead alone in a car on a dark street, in a seedy hotel room, and in the underbrush of a public park. I have treated overdoses in homes, rich and poor, where the patient was found by a loved one. Go on any of these calls, and you will never again consider any user deserving of that fate.

She curls on the couch sobbing. She found her son not breathing when she came home from her midnight shift. He is on the floor now. The fire department first responders do compressions on his bare chest.

The man is lean and muscled with jailhouse tattoos on his arms, chest, and neck. It isn't a stretch to think heroin's the cause. His mother's boyfriend confirms this to us. The man on the floor was a user. They argued about it every day, the boyfriend says, but he kept using. Two torn heroin bags are retrieved from the floor of the bathroom.

We work him for twenty minutes with no response. Asystole throughout. His skin is cool, his pupils fixed and dilated. There is already some stiffening in his jaw. We call the hospital for permission to cease resuscitation. It is granted. We remove the airway, electrodes, and defibrillator pads and place them along with our gloves in the bag the Ambu bag came in.

His mom kneels over him now, kissing his face, her tears falling on his cold skin. "*Vente conmigo, vente conmigo,*" she cries. (Come with me, come with me.) "*No te vayas, no te vayas.*" (Do not go, do not go.) "*Mi niño, mi amor, mi corazon, te quiero.*" (My son, my love, my heart, I love you.) "*Vente conmigo, no te vayas.*"

I stand by his feet holding a clean white sheet. I am motionless.

I attend an opioid symposium where they play a video of a young woman, Daphne Willis, singing a song she wrote about homelessness, addiction, mental illness, and hope. The song is called "Somebody's Someone."[3] As the video plays, many in the audience openly weep.

Plateau

The *Merriam-Webster* online dictionary provides the following definitions of *plateau*:

> plateau (noun): a usually extensive land area having a relatively level surface raised sharply above adjacent land on at least one side.
>
> plateau (verb): to reach a level, period, or condition of stability or maximum attainment.[1]

In 2018 the US health secretary announced that opioid overdose deaths appear to be plateauing across the country. While some states have seen a decrease and others an increase, the overall numbers appear to have slowed after a parabolic rise.[2] The credit for this change can go to harm reduction programs, public health and safety efforts, and community organizations that have worked hard toward finding solutions. Good news certainly, but not cause to disarm. The number of deaths, even if plateauing, is staggering: 52,404 in 2015, 63,632 in 2016, 70,237 in 2017, and 67,367 in 2018.[3] In Connecticut in 2018, we also saw a slight dip in deaths after years of rises, which gave us great hope; those hopes are now dashed, however, with the recent release of 2019

numbers that show the highest total ever, a nearly 20 percent increase over 2018.[4] Many young people, who would otherwise have
had many years of life left, in which to make a family, work, and
contribute to society, vanished long before their time. Many more
will be ensnared by and succumb to this terrible epidemic, particularly as fentanyl deaths continue to rise. *Ensnare* is also a powerful word. Here are its synonyms from the *Merriam-Webster* online
thesaurus: *catch up, enmesh, ensnarl, entangle, entrap, mesh, net,
tangle, trap.*[5]

I attend the Connecticut Bar Association Opioid Conference at
Quinnipiac University School of Law. The conference begins with
a heartbreaking video message from a retired judge, the Honor-
able Anne C. Dranginis, who lost a daughter to opioid overdose
after twelve years of struggling with addiction. She calls her child's
journey into opioids "an innocent entry" and "an impossible exit."
She says that no one is immune. For people who feel "the shame
of addiction," she says, we need to "envelop them with love."[6]

Powerful and true words.

Hartford is quiet early this October. I am involved in a process of
tracking opioid overdoses in our service area, and we witness a lull
in the first half of the month. Overdoses are down 50 percent.
Driving along Park Street, the ever-present users on the nod seem
to have disappeared, as if taken by spaceship. What is going on? I
inquire of neighboring services, ask at the hospitals, and talk to
users on the street. They all report the same things. Overdoses are
way down.

Is it a turning point or a temporary downturn?

Then things start picking up again. The nodders are back. New
brands hit the streets, as well as some oldies: Red Star, Power Hour,
Pray for Death, Fuck You, Power Ball, One Way. Calls for overdoses come in. Naloxone vials come off the shelves. Users have

their respirations restored, with some denying they used, some vowing never to use again, and others choosing to say nothing.

I do ODs three days in a row.

An old man sits slumped on a porch, unconscious. In another world, I am thinking stroke, diabetes, or excessive drinking. His wife, who called 911, sits at the table and shakes her head. "Heroin," she says. "He's at it again." We nudge him and barely get a response. His pupils are pinpoint. His oxygen saturation is 86. He has chronic obstructive pulmonary disease. The level of carbon dioxide in his exhalation is above 70. Along with administering oxygen, we give him just enough naloxone to get his oxygen saturation above 90, his carbon dioxide below 50, and so get him to mumble some answers. Instead of an empty vodka bottle, we find a torn glassine envelope by his chair. A $4 bag of heroin is cheaper than a pint of vodka on the avenue, and the effect is more pleasing. I don't know the relationship between the man and his wife, but I suspect that heroin offers him a form of escape. Today he just caught a bag with a hot spot. At the hospital he is alert enough to admit he snorts a little heroin now and then.

A young man collapses on the sidewalk across the street from the walk-in center. A bystander throws his ice-filled Slurpee on the man's pants. The commotion draws Alex Diaz from the walk-in center with a naloxone injector in hand, a more evidence-based approach than the home remedy of ice in the pants. The young man comes around with some bagging and another 0.4 milligrams of naloxone by IV from us. The crowd of thirty or so all praise each other and EMS for saving another life, while the young man hangs his head in shame as a woman lectures him that this had better be the last time.

The third patient has no human audience for his overdose. No disapproving wife to call 911. No bystander to fill his pants with ice.

He dies alone, his death witnessed only by the skulls on the torn glassine envelopes by his bedside.

Twelve hundred people die of overdose in Connecticut in 2019. One hundred and twenty-three people die of overdose in Hartford, up from ninety-five in 2018 and eighty in 2017.[7] Years ago, a US senator, William Proxmire, had a saying about federal spending: "A million dollars here and a million dollars there, and pretty soon you are talking about real money." Altered for the opioid epidemic, the saying might be this: "A thousand bodies here and a thousand bodies there, and pretty soon you are talking about a real massacre."

State Capitol

I take the day off from work. Instead of putting on my paramedic uniform, I get out my old suit and my one blue tie with a pattern of Charter Oak trees on it. (The Charter Oak was a famous tree in Hartford in the colonial era and early republic.) The tie is the official tie of A Connecticut Party, the party that my old boss Lowell Weicker created for his successful independent run for governor back in 1990. Today, I am returning to the state capitol where I worked for four years between 1991 and 1994. This will not be the first time I have gone back. A number of times over the years I testified before the legislature on bills affecting emergency medical services. I also led a rally at the capitol protesting cuts to the state budget for EMS. Today, I am receiving the 2018 Commissioner of Public Health's Award in recognition of my contributions to pre-hospital care. The award is given once a year, and after twenty-seven years, it is my turn to get it. At the ceremony Commissioner Raul Pino says how much he respects the work I have done on policy while also working each week on the front lines. He mentions my efforts on behalf of the underserved, and then he shakes my hand. While I have always relied on my own internal validation, it is nice to have the career choice I made almost three decades ago publicly acknowledged as a helpful one.

Many of the action items I put on my list after attending the state opioid overdose conference have come to fruition. Working with Ralf Coler and Rich Kamin of the state health department, we have hosted several opioid forums for EMS across the state and created an online training module. The state printed thousands of EMS harm reduction pamphlets that we can give to people. The pamphlet gives advice on using opioids safely, explains how to obtain naloxone, and provides a toll-free number for getting help. Emergency medics now carry non-opioid (and non-addictive) pain management alternatives to morphine and fentanyl, such as Tylenol, ibuprofen, Motrin, and Toradol, so that we can help people with moderate pain without resorting to opioids (which are still best in acute situations for severe pain). We are still working on permitting EMS to leave naloxone with families and are considering a program similar to one started in New Jersey where medics provide a starting dose of buprenorphine to patients who have been revived with naloxone to ease their withdrawal symptoms and dim their cravings, which may make the patients more receptive to getting help in the ED rather than heading right back out to Park for another fix.

Having perhaps the greatest impact is our EMS early warning and surveillance system. It began with a pilot project in Hartford in which my fellow first responders at American Medical Response called in to the Connecticut Poison Control Center after each suspected opioid overdose and answered a series of ten questions, including whether we identified any heroin bags at the scene. After the success of the pilot, the system went statewide. The program, in conjunction with the Overdose Detection and Mapping Application Program, a federal mapping application, provides near-real-time surveillance of the epidemic as well as valuable demographic information about trends. In the first six months of the statewide program, more than three thousand overdoses were tracked and mapped.

June 1, 2019, is a Saturday. In an apartment near Saint Francis Hospital, three people gather to smoke crack. They have only two pipes. While the third user goes into a bedroom to get a third pipe, the first two fire up their bowls. They are unresponsive within moments. A call to 911 brings an ambulance crew to the scene, and they revive the overdosed patients with naloxone. The medics think it strange that the users insist they don't do opioids, only crack. While they are registering the patients at the hospital, another medic brings in a patient who swore he only used crack but also was revived with naloxone. The medics mention this when they call in to poison control. Poison control alerts the state health department to a possible anomaly.

The calls keep coming. By evening there have been nine overdoses in Hartford and two in a neighboring suburb, many of the users claiming only to use crack. Notification is sent out to local harm reduction organizations as well as to city police and health departments. The next two days see a lull, and then on Tuesday, all hell breaks loose. I am sent for an unresponsive person in the north end. I find a man in the driver's seat, head back, mouth open, not breathing, with pinpoint pupils. A bystander says a second person grabbed the man's crack pipe and ran. He responds to naloxone, and in the hospital, he swears to me that he only uses crack. Another medic tells me he responded to a similar call an hour earlier in the same vicinity. On the radio, I hear two other crews clearing scenes with presumptions (of dead patients).

The alarm bells are rung. I stop at Mark's walk-in center and at the needle exchange van. Both places have already mobilized. They spread the word to their clients and pass out fentanyl test strips. They also send out search parties for clients they haven't seen. The next morning, my new partner Cassandra Smith, working an overtime shift, finds a man in rigor mortis sitting in his chair with his crack pipe still in his hand. Another suburban town reports a double overdose by people who say they use only cocaine. While it remains a mystery whether the batch was accidentally contaminated or resulted from a cook deciding to season the mix with fentanyl, the message it sends to all is chilling. No one is safe. Even if you use only crack or cocaine, you need to take precautions, have naloxone available, don't use alone, and call 911 when someone overdoses.

Senator Richard Blumenthal calls a town meeting in Hartford to address the crisis. After the designated speakers, including Mark Jenkins, have spoken, Blumenthal asks if anyone else has anything to share. I remember how my old boss Lowell Weicker used to quote Hubert Humphrey, who told the story of being a young man and being afraid to speak up at a meeting of important people; Humphrey then remembered that it was his job to speak up and to bring the voices of the poor and powerless to the halls of power. I raise my hand and then stand before the gathering. I am no longer a young man, but I can still speak from the heart.

The next day the *Hartford Courant* runs a picture of me addressing the crowd. My hand is raised in the air as I speak. I am animated. I tell the assembly I would rather have users shoot up next to my ambulance than in an alley where we later find them dead because there was no one there to witness their overdose. "The people who use drugs are members of our community," I say, "and they need to be welcomed back home rather than" dispersed.[1]

The epidemic at times makes me think of the opening scene of Homer's *Iliad*, where the Greek general Agamemnon has angered Apollo by stealing the daughter of Apollo's favored priest to be his concubine. In retribution, Apollo rains arrows from the sky that randomly strike down Agamemnon's soldiers. It continues night and day, with no end in sight.

If the opioid epidemic is retaliation for humans having abused a favored drug of the gods, I hope we can find some way to appease them. I don't know if the gods are angry because we had the arrogance to believe we could cure all pain or if they are upset with us because we elevated profit above caring for our fellow human beings. Maybe if we admit, as Agamemnon did, that we were wrong, they will relent. Whereas he was wrong to take the daughter of a priest, we were wrong to take the opium poppy into the laboratory and turn it into profit instead of using it to heal people. Maybe if we can work together to restore balance, the gods will call off the destruction.

We in EMS are not immune to the deaths. The epidemic claims children of two of my coworkers on the ambulance service. A paramedic in another city is injured in an ambulance accident, is prescribed pain pills by a friendly physician, and then sinks into addiction. He is found dead on the job, leaving behind a young wife and child. Having more than twenty-five years in this profession, I know that all of us are always one step away from lying on the stretcher ourselves and looking up into the eyes of someone who does our work and hoping this person shows us mercy.

There is no magic wand to end the killing. Curbing six-month opioid prescriptions will help in the long term, as will advocating non-opioid analgesic alternatives such as ibuprofen and acetaminophen, which studies have shown are just as effective as opioids for treating moderate pain and are certainly safer.[2] Increasing the availability of Suboxone and methadone will help as well. These medications are lifesaving, and we should embrace the idea that, for some, they are as essential as heart, lung, or diabetes medicine.

If taking these medications for the rest of their life enables them to work and support their family and enjoy the experiences that life has to offer, then these medications should be normalized. We have to end the stigma of addiction by recognizing it as a disease and treating it openly. And, above all, we need to advocate fiercely for harm reduction to keep the most vulnerable from falling through the cracks. Harm reduction really just means using common sense: treating people as human beings, treating them like your brother or sister, treating someone like you would want your children treated if you weren't there to protect them. Harm reduction means community naloxone, walk-in centers with needle exchange, safe-injection sites, and even free testing of users' purchased drugs. That way they know what contaminants are in their supply and so can determine which dealers to trust for the cleanest product. And it means giving money directly to these local organizations rather than to multilayered health bureaucracies. We should even consider what Switzerland and England have done, which is to allow certain users access to medical-grade heroin in supervised health clinics.[3] We have to drop the tough-guy stance of incarcerating users and start saving lives by following what has been proven to work. If we give the lost and forsaken confidence and love, if we show them a path to recovery, we may make some headway. If we can stop chasing them into the shadows, where they use alone and unsafely, we can end the deaths.

I sit in the ambulance and watch gaunt young men and women walk up Park Street to meet their dealers. It is a hot day, and I have a cooler of bottled water and some oranges and apples. I hand out some to passersby and ask how their day is going. We share information about the brands on the street. I pass on the warning to be careful of a brand stamped "Kit Kat," which has made a number of users sick. If they are going to use Red Devil, do a tester shot first. It is potent. I watch one young man eat an apple like he hasn't eaten in a month.

Later that afternoon we respond to an overdose on Hudson Street by a dumpster. Fire department first responders gave the man 4 milligrams of naloxone. They mention that he had already been Narcaned once by a passerby. The man comes around and vomits. He denies that he used drugs, but in the ambulance, he admits to using Red Devil. He is from Simsbury and is only twenty-three, although he looks much younger. He says he got addicted to pain pills following a skiing accident. He got out of rehab last week. I hand him a pamphlet that has the number of the twenty-four-hour opioid hotline and explains where he can obtain naloxone. I give him a talk on harm reduction and tell him about where to get clean needles. I tell him about the dangers of fentanyl and advise him never to use alone.

"Why are you being so nice to me," he says. "I'm a scumbag."

I explain how my views have changed, how I now understand that addiction is a brain disease and not a character flaw.

"You should talk to my parents," he says.

I see Chloe. She is now living behind the strip mall at 1200 Park. Last week she got beaten up by a man who'd given her a ride. She said he had no money to pay her for her services, so he slugged her. Her eye looks much better today than it did last week. She says she went to rehab for four days but wasn't quite ready to commit to it. I'm going to make it one of these times, she says. I give her an apple and four dollars because I can see she is not doing well.

"I'd like to meet you one day when I'm done with all of this," she says.

"That would be nice," I say.

What would you do if you found out that one of your loved ones was addicted to opioids and had lost their way? What would you hope another person would do for them while you lie awake at night wondering where they are, or if they are even still alive? Do you pray for kindness in the world?

This battle may never be won, but as long as we can save one person or keep another alive for a year longer, or maybe even just to see another sunrise, it is worth fighting.

Another 911 call comes in for an overdose. We respond.

Epilogue

Kelly disappears, and weeks go by with no sight of her. I finally see Jackson, her boyfriend's cousin, and he tells us that Tom got out of jail and is looking fit. He took Kelly with him down to Middletown, where he is in a rehab program. A few months later, Jackson updates me. He thinks they are living in New Jersey with Tom's mom. I like to think of them living in a small house, with Tom coming home from work in a shirt and tie and Kelly cooking a meal that warms the house. And they are, for at least that night, safe from the temptations that lurk just streets away.

Veronica disappears for months. I worry when I hear word that her sister was seen looking for her. Through my friends at the needle exchange van, I finally learn that she returned to northwestern Connecticut, but they are uncertain whether she is living with her sister or with someone else. Then another medic tells me he treated her for an OD on Park Street. A nurse at the hospital tells me she was in the ED in cardiac arrest, but they got her back. She has no more details than that. I look each day for her, but she has vanished again. Months go by. No one has seen her. Then one day we are parked across from Pope Park, and all of a sudden she is standing right in front of me with a big smile. I get out of the ambulance and lift her up in the air and give her a hug. She tells me her tale.

She went to the ED one night, not even high but not feeling well. She left after an hour because no one would see her, and she started to get drug sick. Then an ambulance responded, and the crew blasted her with Narcan and made her violently sick. "I'm tired of peeling your ass off the street," the paramedic told her. (I find this greatly upsetting.) When she went into the ED, the nurse declared, "Her again! She was just here!" In the ED, Veronica went into cardiac arrest, twice. She needed an emergency pacemaker and then surgery for a heart valve replacement. This was the third time she has had one owing to endocarditis.

Veronica shows me the fresh scar on her chest. Despite the way she was treated, she is thankful to the system for saving her life, she says now. She was at the hospital for two months, and they made a cake for her when she was finally released. She says she doesn't want to be a disappointment to those who have cared for her and care about her, but she doesn't think she will ever be able to stop using permanently. The power heroin has over her is too great.

Inez is still out in front of the bakery every day. Sometimes she is sweeping the sidewalk or washing cars for a few extra bucks. Other times she squats in a small shaded corner, watching the street. When I see her, I say to her, "You want two dollars, or you want me to buy you some lunch?"

"Two dollars," she says.

I give her the two dollars and then go into El Mercado and come out with a bag containing an alcapurria (a fritter with meat inside) and a Champagne cola, which I hand to her. "You said you wanted lunch, right?"

"Thank you, baby," she says. "See you tomorrow. Be safe."

I am working with a fill-in partner, who questions whether giving a heroin user money is, effectively, enabling drug use.

"Her life is hard enough," I say. "A little kindness can't be a bad thing. At least she knows she's not alone."

Gloria vanishes. So does Mickey. No word of either from anyone.

Randy, the young man who argued with his mother in the plaza, is found dead in a motel south of the city. Lying next to him on the bed are a needle and torn heroin bags branded "Scorpion."

Luke hangs out outside McDonald's, where customers might give him some change as he sits with his head down, reading a book. I stop by and give him $5, and he gives me another lesson on spinning a basketball on my finger. He says I am getting better. I ask him if he played in his younger days. He says he was a street baller but was always getting into too much trouble to play on a team. He says I might not be seeing him much longer. He and a buddy are considering starting a handyman business with the help of a local Christian organization. Then one day, he is gone. I have a picture that my daughter took of me spinning a basketball with a Harlem Globetrotter when the team came to town. I want to show it to Luke so that he can be proud of his pupil. I worry, though, that if I see him again, it will be because he is back on the street. Maybe one day he'll pull into McDonald's in a truck with "Luke's Construction" written on the side, and we will sit inside the restaurant together, and he will tell me of his recovery and new life.

Chloe stumbles down the street. Her hand is over her face. "I'm sick of living like this," she says, and I am worried she has been hit again. No, she says, her eye is infected. It is red and oozing pus.

"You need to get that looked at," I say.

"Can't I just wash it out?"

"No, we can take you to the ER."

"I'll go with you," she says. "But I'm really sick." I give her four dollars. It is a Sunday morning, and the dealers aren't out yet. "Come back for me in an hour," she says, "and I'll go with you."

No matter how many times this scene plays out between us, I remain hopeful that today will be the day she says yes to rehab. I think about how I can make my pitch. We can take her to Saint Francis, where she can get on Suboxone. They'll find her a bed somewhere, tend to her eye, and heal her abscesses. Maybe this time will be the charm for her. Maybe she'll decide to become an addiction counselor and use her real-world experience to help others. We go on some calls, and after each one, we drive back to Park Street. But Chloe is nowhere to be found. Two weeks go by with no sign of her. I worry about her, alone in the world.

On my day off, I am driving my daughter to a softball game on a route that takes us through Hartford. I turn right onto Park Terrace and notice that a late-model Subaru ahead of me has its hazard lights flashing and is pulled over at the edge of the park. Other cars honk at the temporary traffic congestion. A middle-aged woman in a yellow dress and polished white shoes walks to a bench where a younger woman lies. I recognize the younger woman as Chloe. Her face is battered and bruised, and she looks sick. The woman in the dress sits down on the bench and gently takes Chloe's head into her lap. The woman has a water bottle in her hand. She raises the water to Chloe's lips, and Chloe drinks.

$, 1, 1 of 1, 4 Way, 9 Plus, 12 Monkeys, 23 Jordan, 24-7, 64, 69, 100%, 121, 127, 2017, A+, Adidas, AK-47, Alias, Alien Rock, All the Way Down, Always Good, Amazing, Arm and Hammer, Atomic, Attitude Adjustment (Fuck You), Avatar, Avengers, Back Off, Bad Boys, Bad Bunny, Balmier, Bass Pass, Bat, Batman, Beat Street, Be Cool, Best Buy, Big Apple, Big Doodle, Bingo 9, Biohazard, Birthday Cake, Black Devil, Black Heat, Black Ice, Black Jack, Black Out, Black Panther, Black Rose, Black Sunday, Black Widow, Blaze, Block Party, Blow, Blue Apple, Boo!, Bugatti, Bugs Bunny, Butterfly, Buzz Off, Call of Duty, Camera, Campfire, Candy Cane, Cartel, Cartier, Casino, Casper, Certified Bitch, Check, Check Plus, Cherry, Chicken Curry 30, Chief, Chinese Letters, Chipotle, Chosen Few, Cobra, Coca-Cola, Come Back, Compton, Connecticut, Cool Water, Copy, Crazy Monkey, Crown, Crunch Time, Cum Up, Dance, Danger, Danger Zone, Day Dose, Dead Flower, Dead Like Me, Dead Man, Dead Men, Denny's, Design, Designer, Devil, Devil Around, Dice, Diesel, Dinamita, Dinosaur, Dirty Money, Dirty Sprite, Dog, Donald Trump, Donkey Kong, Don Season, Don't Front, Down Time, Dream Chaser, Dubai, Ducati, Eagle, Eiffel Tower, El Chapo, El Loco, Emerald City, Empire, EZ Pass, Face, Faces, Faded, Fairy, Fantastic, Fast Lane, Fastrack, Fat Turkey, Faxed, Ferrari, The Finals, Fire, Fireball, Firework, Five Star, The Flash, Flower, Focus, Foxy, French Montana, Friday the 13th, Froggie, Frown, Fruit Punch, Fuck You, Fury, Future, Game of Thrones, Gas Face, Gas Monkey, Gatorade, Get Lucky, Giraffe, G.O.A.T., Golden State, Good and Plenty, Good 4 You, Good Work, Gorilla, Got Fire, Goya, Grade A, Great Job, Great Whites, Green Dragon, Green Eyes, Green Is Good, Grey Goose, Gucci, Gummy Bear, Guns, H, Hall Pass, Happy, Hard Ten, Harley-Davidson, Head Games, Headphones, Head Trauma, Heartbreak, Heaven Hell, Hello Kitty, Hennessy, Hess, High Life, High Power, High Time, High Voltage, Holiday Season, Hook Me Up, Horsepower, Hot Sauce, Howl, Hulk, HY, Hype, I Got Fire, I'll Be Back, Illuminati, Impac, Indian Chief, Intercontinentals, It, It's Hot, Jackpot,

Jason and Freddy, Jcull Candy, JFK (New York, NY), Johnny Walker, Joker, Joker 2 Go, Jungle, Jungle Killer, Just for You, Kamikaze, KD, Kermit, KFC, KickStart, Kid Face, Kill Bill, Killer Clowns, Killer Instinct, Killing Season, Killing Time, Kim, King, King of Death, Kiss, Kiss Me, Kit Kat, Kmart, KO, Kool-Aid, KTM, Lady Bug, Lake of the Dead, Lamborghini, Latin Power, La-Z-Boy, Level Up, Life Saver, Light Bulb, Lizard, Louis Vuitton, Lucky 7, Magic, Magic City, Magoo, Man Down, Martini, Marvin the Martian, The Mechanic, Merchant of Death, MGM, Miami, Middle Finger, Mind Craft, Mind Eraser, Mojo, Money Bags, Money Talks, Most Wanted, Mula, Music, Mustang, Need for Speed, Nelly Rider, New Arrival, New High Score: Ultimate Level, Newport, Newports, New World, NFL, Nick at Nite, Night Owl, Nike, Nirvana, Nite Nite, No Cap, No Evil, No Stopping, No Way Out, Oh My God, OK, Old School, Oliver Queen, OMG, On Demand, One Dab, One to Go, One Way, OTF, Out of Stock, Pacquiao, Paid, Panda, Panther, Paradise, Party Time, Passion, Past Due, Patron, Peace Sign, Peter Rabbit, Phat Batch, Pirate, Pirates, Pirate Ship, Playboy, Pokemon, Poker, Polka Dot, Polo, Pooty Tang, Pound for Pound, Power, Power Grip, Power House, Power Punch, Power Shack, Predator, Present, Pride, Pringles, Processed, PRV, Public Enemy, Puma, The Purge, Purple Rein, Race Horse, Racetrack, Ralph Lauren, Reaper, Red Bull, Red Devils, Red Fox, Red Line, Red Lion, Red Star, Remy, Ride or Die, RKO, Rockstar, ROC Nation, ROL, Rolex, Rolls Royce, RR, Samsung, Satan, Satyr, Sazon, Scorpion, ShakaZulu, Shine, Ship's Wheel, Shooting Star, Sin City, Skittles, Skull and Bones, Sky High, Sling Shot, Slipper, Smart Car, Smiley Face, Smiley Star, Smurfs, Snake, Snapchat, Snapple, Snowman, Sony, Soul Survivor, Space Jam, Spade, Spartan Helmet, Speed Limit 50, Spider, Spider Web, Spring Break, Sprite, Star, Stars, Stranger Danger, Strike Dead, Strong Arm, Summertime, Super Bee, Super Bowl, Super Bowl 50, Superman, Super Mario, Supreme, SweetHeart, Taco Bell, Takeover, Tak'n Over, Team, Tesla, Thanks, Think Green, Thor, Thumbs Up, TKO, TMT, Top Gun, Toro, Trump, The Truth, TS, Tunnel Vision, UCONN, Unforgiven, Universe, Uno, Upside Down, USA, USA Power, USA Skull, Vamp, Venom, Venom H2O, Versace, Vigilante, Vigilante 13, W2, Walking Dead, Wassupp!!!, Way to Go, Wendy's, White Castle, White Sand, WiFi, Wi-Fight, Wildcat, Wild Fire, Witch Doctor, Wolf, World Star, Worldwide, Wow, X, XXX, You First, Zika, Zika Virus.

ACKNOWLEDGMENTS

I would like to thank Rich Kamin, the EMS medical director at UConn John Dempsey Hospital, who has been a great friend and who allowed me to spend time on EMS-oriented approaches to the opioid epidemic, and Ralf Coler, who, as the head of Connecticut's Office of Emergency Medical Services, has been a strong supporter of a central role for EMS in fighting the epidemic. I would also like to thank Dr. Steven Wolf of Saint Francis Hospital and Medical Center for his commitment to improving care for opioid users and for being a great medical control physician for the paramedics at American Medical Response in Hartford. I would like to thank Chris Chaplin and Brandon Bartell, operations managers at American Medical Response, for their support, as well as supervisor Jeremy Dumas.

I would like to thank my partners, Jerry Sneed, Bryan Sabin, Cassandra Smith, and Chris Trembley, for tolerating my obsessions: from looking for heroin bags, to driving slowly down Park Street, to seeking out and checking on the people we came to know. And thanks to the young paramedics we trained, Dan Fraczek, Tom Palomba, Amanda Longo, Andrew Eccles, Daniel Hammersmith, Rachael Kenyon, and Katherine Eaton, who have all become not only great paramedics but also budding harm reductionists.

I would like to thank people in the harm reduction community who welcomed me and showed me the way, including Mark Jenkins, Shawn Lang, Sarah Howroyd, Alixe Dittmore, Norm LeBlanc, LaToya Tyson, Mike Grace, Sue Clark, and Alex Diaz.

Thanks to Kelsey Opozda, Sarah Ali, and Bob Lawler of the New England High Intensity Drug Trafficking Area and Steve Citta of the Hartford Police Department for their insights into the epidemic.

Thanks to Charles McKay, Suzanne Doyon, Kathy Hart, Elizabeth Laska, and all the specialists at the Connecticut Poison Control Center for their help and friendship. Thanks to Rob Fuller at UConn Health ED.

I would like to thank my great and loyal agent, Jane Dystel, for her tireless support and guidance over the years and for not giving up on this book. Thanks also to Miriam Goderich at Dystel, Goderich & Bourrett LLC for her help with my writing.

Thank you to Robin Coleman for acquiring my manuscript and for his excellent suggestions for improving the book. Thank you to Robert Brown, who did a fantastic job of copyediting the manuscript, and to others at Johns Hopkins University Press for their creativity and efforts on behalf of this book. Thanks also to the anonymous peer reviewers for their important thoughts.

Most of all I would like to thank the people of Hartford who shared their stories with me and helped me better understand the forces behind the epidemic and see the goodness and hope in every human being.

Prologue

1. Lawrence Scholl, Puja Seth, Mbabazi Kariisa, Nana Wilson, and Grant Baldwin, "Drug and Opioid-Involved Overdose Deaths—United States, 2013–2017," *Morbidity and Mortality Weekly Report* 67, nos. 51–52 (2019): 1419–27.

Chapter 1. Hartford, Connecticut, 1995

1. Maxine Bernstein, "Homicide Rate Fell in Hartford in '95," *Hartford Courant*, January 1, 1996; George Coppolo and Ryan O'Neil, *Murder Rates in Connecticut and Other States and Certain Cities.* OLR Research Report, September 14, 2005. https://www.cga.ct.gov/2005/rpt/2005-R-0639.htm.

2. Evelyn Nieves, "A Violent Battle of Wills Besieges Hartford," *Hartford Courant*, December 24, 1994.

3. Susan Campbell and Frances Grandy Taylor, "A Year Later, Death of Marcelina Delgado Galvanizes Community," *Hartford Courant*, March 26, 1995; Jenna Carlesso, "20 Years Ago, Shooting Death Drove City's War on Gang Violence," *Hartford Courant*, October 28, 2014.

Chapter 2. Park Street, 2016

1. Dave Collins, "Gangs Aren't Wearing Colors Anymore," *Business Insider*, September 16, 2014. https://www.businessinsider.com/gangs-arent-wearing-colors-anymore-2014-9.

Chapter 3. Antipathy

1. "What Is Moral Injury," The Moral Injury Project, Syracuse University, n.d. http://moralinjuryproject.syr.edu/about-moral-injury/.

2. "Weymouth Firefighter Suspended for Facebook Post about Narcan," CBS Boston, February 1, 2016. https://boston.cbslocal.com/2016/02/01/weymouth-firefighter-facebook-post-narcan-addicts/.

3. Brian MacQuarrie, "Weymouth Suspends Firefighter over Social Media Post," *Boston Globe*, February 1, 2016. https://www.bostonglobe.com/metro/2016/02/01/weymouth-fire-chief-investigating-social-media-post

-that-allegedly-disparaged-heroin-addicts/akRkLfMRR8CDBJ5Lrl92EN
/story.html.

4. "Narcan," Law Enforcement Rant (discussion board), August 18,
2017. http://lerant.proboards.com/thread/8197/narcan.

5. Cody Shepard, "State Police Dispatcher from Brockton Suspended
over Facebook Comments," *Taunton (MA) Daily Gazette*, March 29, 2018.
https://www.tauntongazette.com/news/20180328/state-police-dispatcher
-from-brockton-suspended-over-facebook-comments.

6. Rebecca Lurye, "Hartford Police Officer under Investigation for
'Derogatory' Social Media Post," *Hartford Courant*, October 3, 2019.

7. "The Fastest Way to Sober Up Heroin Addicts," YouTube, December 13, 2016. https://youtu.be/Q_aajvrh7AE.

8. Cleve R. Wootson Jr., "Why This Ohio Sheriff Refuses to Let His
Deputies Carry Narcan to Reverse Overdoses," *Washington Post*, July 8,
2017. https://www.washingtonpost.com/news/to-your-health/wp/2017/07
/08/an-ohio-countys-deputies-could-reverse-heroin-overdoses-the-sheriff
-wont-let-them/?utm_term=.15965072409e.

9. Cleve R. Wootson Jr., "One Politician's Solution to the Overdose
Problem: Let Addicts Die," *Washington Post*, June 30, 2017. https://www
.washingtonpost.com/news/to-your-health/wp/2017/06/28/a-council
-members-solution-to-his-ohio-towns-overdose-problem-let-addicts-die
/?utm_term=.8ccae159333b.

10. Peter Canning, *Paramedic: On the Front Lines of Medicine* (New York:
Ballantine Books, 1998), 255–56.

Chapter 4. Empathy

1. *Facing Addiction in America: The Surgeon General's Report on Alcohol,
Drugs, and Health* (Washington, DC: US Department of Health and Human
Services, 2016). https://addiction.surgeongeneral.gov/sites/default/files
/surgeon-generals-report.pdf.

2. Chad Newland, Erich Barber, Monique Rose, and Amy Young,
"Survey Reveals Alarming Rates of EMS Provider Stress and Thoughts of
Suicide," *Journal of Emergency Medical Services*, September 28, 2015.
https://www.jems.com/articles/print/volume-40/issue-10/features
/survey-reveals-alarming-rates-of-ems-provider-stress-and-thoughts-of
-suicide.html.

Chapter 5. Addiction

1. "City of East Liverpool, Ohio," Facebook, September 8, 2016.
https://www.facebook.com/cityofeastliverpool/posts/879927698809767.

2. "What Is Addiction?," American Psychiatric Association. https://
www.psychiatry.org/patients-families/addiction/what-is-addiction.

3. *Public Policy Statement: Short Definition of Addiction*, American Society of Addiction Medicine, 2011. https://www.asam.org/docs/default -source/publications/asam-news-archives/vol26-3.pdf?sfvrsn=0.

4. Donna De La Cruz, "Opioids May Interfere with Parenting Instincts, Study Finds," *New York Times*, October 13, 2016. https://www.nytimes.com /2016/10/13/well/family/opioids-may-interfere-with-parenting-instincts -study-finds.html.

5. "Treatment and Recovery," National Institute on Drug Abuse, last updated July 2018. https://www.drugabuse.gov/publications/drugs-brains -behavior-science-addiction/treatment-recovery.

6. *Facing Addiction in America: The Surgeon General's Report on Alcohol, Drugs, and Health* (Washington, DC: US Department of Health and Human Services, 2016).

7. Richard Miech, Lloyd Johnston, Patrick M. O'Malley, Katherine M. Keyes, and Kennon Heard, "Prescription Opioids in Adolescence and Future Opioid Misuse," *Pediatrics* 136, no. 5 (2015): e1169–e1177. doi:10.1542/peds.2015-1364.

8. "Chasing the Dragon," Urban Dictionary, December 29, 2004. https://www.urbandictionary.com/define.php?term=Chasing%20the%20 dragon.

Chapter 6. Stigma

1. *Merriam-Webster*, s.v. "stigma (*n.*)," accessed August 18, 2019. https://www.merriam-webster.com/dictionary/stigma.

2. *Understanding Drug-Related Stigma and Discrimination: Tools for Better Practice and Social Change* [PowerPoint slideshow] (New York: Harm Reduction Coalition, 2010). https://harmreduction.org/wp-content /uploads/2012/02/Slides.pdf.

3. *Understanding Drug-Related Stigma: Tools for Better Practice and Social Change* [participant workbook] (New York: Harm Reduction Coalition, n.d.), 10. https://harmreduction.org/wp-content/uploads/2012 /02/participant-workbook.pdf.

4. Brendan Murphy, "4 Factors That Add to Stigma Surrounding Opioid-Use Disorder," American Medical Association, September 13, 2018. https://www.ama-assn.org/delivering-care/opioids/4-factors-add-stigma -surrounding-opioid-use-disorder; Michael P. Botticelli, Memorandum to the Heads of Executive Departments and Agencies; Subject: Changing Federal Terminology regarding Substance Use and Substance Use Disorders (Washington, DC: Office of National Drug Control Policy, January 9, 2017). https:// www.whitehouse.gov/sites/whitehouse.gov/files/images/Memo%20-%20 Changing%20Federal%20Terminology%20Regrading%20Substance%20 Use%20and%20Substance%20Use%20Disorders.pdf.

5. William L. White, "The Rhetoric of Recovery Advocacy: An Essay on the Power of Language," in *Let's Go Make Some History: Chronicles of the New Addiction Recovery Advocacy Movement* (Washington, DC: Johnson Institute and Faces and Voices of Recovery, 2006), 37–76, p. 2 in http://www.williamwhitepapers.com/pr/2001RhetoricofRecoveryAdvocacy.pdf.

Chapter 7. Withdrawal and Relapse

1. Scott G. Weiner, Olesya Baker, Dana Bernson, and Jeremiah D. Schuur, "One-Year Mortality of Patients after Emergency Department Treatment for Nonfatal Opioid Overdose," *Annals of Emergency Medicine* 75, no. 1 (2020): 13–17.

2. S. F. J. Clarke, P. I. Dargan, and A. L. Jones, "Naloxone in Opioid Poisoning: Walking the Tightrope," *Emergency Medicine Journal* 22 (2005): 612–16.

3. Michael W. Willman, David B. Liss, Evan S. Schwarz, and Michael E. Mullins, "Do Heroin Overdose Patients Require Observation after Receiving Naloxone?," *Clinical Toxicology* 55, no. 2 (2017): 81–87.

4. Brendan Saloner and Shankar Karthikeyan, "Changes in Substance Abuse Treatment Use among Individuals with Opioid Use Disorders in the United States, 2004–2013," *JAMA* 314, no. 14 (2015): 1515–17.

5. Christopher M. Jones, Melinda Campopiano, Grant Baldwin, and Elinore McCance-Katz, "National and State Treatment Need and Capacity for Opioid Agonist Medication-Assisted Treatment," *American Journal of Public Health* 105 (2015): e55–e63.

6. Peter Canning, Charles McKay, Suzanne Doyon, Elizabeth Laska, Katherine Hart, and Richard Kamin, "Coordinated Surveillance of Opioid Overdoses in Hartford, Connecticut: A Pilot Project," *Connecticut Medicine* 83, no. 6 (2019): 293–99.

7. Sonia Tagliareni, "Relapse Triggers," Drug Rehab.com, May 31, 2018. https://www.drugrehab.com/recovery/triggers/.

Chapter 8. Heartache

1. Homer, *The Odyssey*, translated by Robert Fagles and annotated and introduced by Bernard Knox (New York: Viking, 1996), book 9.

2. Alfred Lord Tennyson, "The Lotos-eaters," Poetry Foundation. https://www.poetryfoundation.org/poems/45364/the-lotos-eaters.

3. "Origins and History of Opium," Herb Museum, 1994. http://www.herbmuseum.ca/content/origins-and-history-opium.

4. "Opioid Addiction 2016 Facts & Figures," American Society of Addiction Medicine. https://www.asam.org/docs/default-source/advocacy/opioid-addiction-disease-facts-figures.pdf.

5. "Economic Toll of Opioid Crisis in U.S. Exceeded $1 Trillion Since 2001," Altarum, December 6, 2018. https://altarum.org/news/economic -toll-opioid-crisis-us-exceeded-1-trillion-2001.

6. Luke Davies, *Candy* (New York: Ballantine Books, 1977).

7. The following is a flyer announcing the event in Bristol, Connecticut: "2019 CT Opioid & Prescription Drug Overdose Prevention Conference." https://portal.ct.gov/-/media/DPH/Injury-Prevention/2019-CT-Opioid -and-Prescription-Drug-Overdose-Prev-Conference.pdf?la=en.

8. N'dea Yancey-Bragg, "Columbine School Shooting Survivor Austin Eubanks Found Dead," *USA Today*, May 19, 2019. https://www.usatoday .com/story/news/nation/2019/05/19/columbine-school-shooting-survivor -austin-eubanks-found-dead/3732079002/.

9. Dave Altimari, "Columbine and Addiction Survivor Austin Eubanks Made His Last Speech at a Connecticut Opioid Conference. He Was Found Dead in Colorado Last Weekend," *Hartford Courant*, May 20, 2019.

Chapter 9. Pain Control

1. "Purdue Pharma OxyContin Commercial," YouTube, posted September 22, 2016. https://www.youtube.com/watch?v=Er78Dj5hyeI.

2. Martin Booth, *Opium: A History* (New York: St. Martin's Griffin, 1999), chapter 5.

3. Barry Meir, "In Guilty Plea, OxyContin Maker to Pay $600 Million," *New York Times*, May 10, 2007.

4. Institute of Medicine, *Relieving Pain in America: A Blueprint for Transforming Prevention, Care, Education, and Research* (Washington, DC: National Academies Press, 2011).

5. American Pain Association, https://painassociation.org/.

6. Christine Clara McEachin, Joseph Thomas McDermott, and Robert Swor, "Few Emergency Medical Services Patients with Lower-Extremity Fractures Receive Prehospital Analgesia," *Prehospital Emergency Care* 6, no. 4 (2002): 406–10.

7. Stephen H. Thomas and Sanjay Shewakramani, "Prehospital Trauma Analgesia," *Journal of Emergency Medicine* 35, no. 1 (2008): 47–57.

8. James Ducharme, Sharon E. Mace, and Michael F. Murphy, *Pain Management and Sedation: Emergency Department Management* (New York: McGraw-Hill, 2006).

9. R. Mackenzie, "Analgesia and Sedation," *Journal of the Royal Army Medical Corps* 146 (2000): 117–27.

10. Jane Porter and Hershel Jick, "Addiction Rare in Patients Treated with Narcotics," *New England Journal of Medicine* 302, no. 2 (1980): 123.

11. Sam Allis Boston, "Less Pain, More Gain," *Time*, June 24, 2001.

12. Pamela T. M. Leung, Erin M. Macdonald, Matthew B. Stanbrook, and Irfan A. Dhalla, "A 1980 Letter on the Risk of Opioid Addiction," *New England Journal of Medicine* 376 (2017): 2194–95.

13. Clifford Allbutt, "On the Abuse of Hypodermic Injections of Morphia," *Practitioner* 5, no. 30 (December 1870): 327–31.

14. Deirdre Shesgreen, Jayne O'Donnell, and Terry DeMio, "How Drug Company Money Turned Patient Groups into 'Cheerleaders for Opioids,'" *Springfield News-Leader*, February 12, 2018.

15. Susan Morse, "CMS, Joint Commission Pressed to Change Policies That Promote Opioid Pain Medicine Overuse," *Healthcare Finance News*, April 14, 2016. https://www.healthcarefinancenews.com/news/cms-joint -commission-pressed-change-policies-promote-opioid-pain-medicine -overuse.

16. Christopher M. Jones and Vanila M. Singh, "Advancing the Practice of Pain Management under the HHS Opioid Strategy," US Department of Health and Human Services, November 1, 2017. https://www.hhs.gov/blog /2017/11/01/advancing-the-practice-of-pain-management-under-the-hhs -opioid-strategy.html.

17. Thomas Sullivan, "Senators Grassley and Wyden Expand Their Opioid Investigation to Tax-Exempt Organizations," *Policy & Medicine*, July 10, 2019. https://www.policymed.com/2019/07/senators-grassley-and -wyden-expand-their-opioid-investigation-to-tax-exempt-organizations .html.

18. Damian McNamara, "American Pain Society Officially Shuttered," *Medscape*, July 2, 2019. https://www.medscape.com/viewarticle/915141 ?nlid=130518_5322&src=WNL_mdplsnews_190705_mscpedit_wir&uac =123576PT&spon=17&impID=2019552&faf=1.

19. "Today's Heroin Epidemic Infographics," Centers for Disease Control and Prevention, last reviewed July 7, 2015. https://www.cdc.gov /vitalsigns/heroin/infographic.html.

20. Kevin E. Vowles, Mindy L. McEntee, Peter Siyahhan Julnes, Tessa Frohe, John P. Ney, and David N. van der Goes, "Rates of Opioid Misuse, Abuse, and Addiction in Chronic Pain: A Systematic Review and Data Synthesis," *Pain* 156, no. 4 (2015): 569–76. doi:10.1097/01.j.pain .0000460357.01998.fi.

21. "Opioid Painkiller Prescribing Infographic," Centers for Disease Control and Prevention, last reviewed July 1, 2014. https://www.cdc.gov /vitalsigns/opioid-prescribing/infographic.html.

22. National Institute on Drug Abuse, "Connecticut Opioid Summary," NIDA, revised March 2019. https://www.drugabuse.gov/drugs-abuse /opioids/opioid-summaries-by-state/connecticut-opioid-summary.

23. Anuj Shah, Corey J. Hayes, and Bradley C. Martin, "Characteristics of Initial Prescription Episodes and Likelihood of Long-Term Opioid Use—United States, 2006–2015, *Morbidity and Mortality Weekly Report* 66, no. 10 (2017): 265–69. doi:http://dx.doi.org/10.15585/mmwr.mm6610a1.

24. Nick Wing, "DEA Cutting Production of Prescription Opioids by 25 Percent in 2017," *HuffPost*, January 3, 2017. https://www.huffpost.com /entry/dea-cutting-prescription-opioids_n_57f50078e4b03254526297bd.

25. John Temple, *American Pain: How a Young Felon and His Ring of Doctors Unleashed America's Deadliest Drug Epidemic* (Guilford, CT: Lyons Press, 2016).

26. Barry Meier, *Pain Killer: A "Wonder" Drug's Trail of Addiction and Death* (Emmaus, PA: Rodale, 2003).

27. Lindsey Bever, "A Town of 3,200 Was Flooded with Nearly 21 Million Pain Pills as Addiction Crisis Worsened, Lawmakers Say," *Washington Post*, January 31, 2018.

28. Jenn Abelson, Andrew Ba Tran, Beth Reinhard, and Aaron C. Davis, "As Overdoses Soared, Nearly 35 Billion Opioids—Half of Distributed Pills—Handled by 15 Percent of Pharmacies," *Washington Post*, August 12, 2019.

29. John Temple, "DEA Secretly OKs Killer Quantities of Oxy and Morphine," *Daily Beast*, October 21, 2015. https://www.thedailybeast.com /dea-secretly-oks-killer-quantities-of-oxy-and-morphine.

30. Lydia Ramsey, "Explosive '60 Minutes' Investigation Finds Congress and Drug Companies Worked to Cripple DEA's Ability to Fight Opioid Abuse," *Business Insider*, October 16, 2017. https://www.business insider.com/60-minutes-drug-industry-worked-against-dea-fight-opioid -epidemic-investigation-2017-10.

31. "The Numbers behind America's Heroin Epidemic," *New York Times*, October 30, 2015.

32. National Institute on Drug Abuse, "Overdose Death Rates," NIDA, January 29, 2019. https://www.drugabuse.gov/related-topics/trends -statistics/overdose-death-rates.

33. National Drug Intelligence Center, "Connecticut Drug Threat Assessment," July 2002. https://www.justice.gov/archive/ndic/pubs07 /997/997p.pdf.

Chapter 10. Kelly and Veronica

1. Carol Glatz, "Don't Worry How It's Spent, Always Give Homeless a Handout, Pope Says," *Catholic News Service*, April 28, 2017. https://www .catholicnews.com/services/englishnews/2017/dont-worry-how-its-spent -always-give-homeless-a-handout-pope-says.cfm.

Chapter 11.   Opioid Conference

1.   *Hearings before the Select Committee on Presidential Campaign Activities of the United States Senate: Ninety-Third Congress, First Session; Watergate and Related Activities, Phase I, June 27, 28, 29, and July 10, 1973, book 4* (Washington, DC: US Government Printing Office, 1973), 1504. Available from the Internet Archive, https://archive.org/details/presidential camp04unit/page/1504/mode/2up.

2.   *The Connecticut Opioid Response Initiative* (strategic plan), October 5, 2016. http://ghhrc.org/wp-content/uploads/2016/10/CORE_CT_Opioid _REsponse_Initiative_100516.pdf.

Chapter 12.   Harm Reduction

1.   Department of Mental Health and Addiction Services, "New Program Connects Overdose Victims to Recovery Coaches" (news release), April 26, 2017. https://www.ct.gov/dmhas/cwp/view.asp?q=592406.

2.   *Fentanyl Test Strip Pilot* (report), Harm Reduction Coalition, February 18, 2018. https://harmreduction.org/issue-area/overdose-prevention -issue-area/fentanyl-test-strip-pilot/.

3.   Maia Szalavitz, "Dan Bigg Is a Harm-Reduction Pioneer and His Overdose Doesn't Change That," *Vice*, October 24, 2018. https://www.vice .com/en_us/article/7x3yag/dan-bigg-overdose-harm-reduction.

4.   Tessie Castillo, "In Memory of Dan Bigg, Harm Reduction Godfather," *Medium*, August 31, 2018. https://medium.com/@tswopecastillo/in -memory-of-dan-bigg-harm-reduction-godfather-ed0abaa09b1d.

Chapter 13.   Fentanyl

1.   Edmund Mahony, "Stalking a 'Serial Killer' Narcotic from Boston to Wichita," *Hartford Courant*, February 23, 1993. https://www.courant.com /news/connecticut/hc-xpm-1993-02-23-0000105550-story.html.

2.   "NYC Police Find 280 Bags of Designer Drug, Study Possible Link to Drug Deaths," AP News, February 5, 1991. https://www.apnews.com/33db 80e67e3baea5c84efb1220350f7d.

3.   *Fentanyl: A Briefing Guide for First Responders* (Washington, DC: Drug Enforcement Administration, n.d.). https://www.nvfc.org/wp -content/uploads/2018/03/Fentanyl-Briefing-Guide-for-First-Responders .pdf.

4.   "Fentanyl," Wikipedia, last edited on March 8, 2020. https://en.wiki pedia.org/wiki/Fentanyl.

5.   Ethan O. Bryson and Jeffrey H. Silverstein, "Addiction and Substance Abuse in Anesthesiology," *Anesthesiology* 109, no. 5, (2008): 905–17. doi:10.1097/ALN.0b013e3181895bc1.

6. Karen S. Sibert, "Why This Anesthesiologist Says 'No' to Fentanyl," KevinMD.com, October 18, 2017. https://www.kevinmd.com/blog/2017/10/anesthesiologist-says-no-fentanyl.html.

7. Will Maddox, "UT Southwestern's Response to Nurses' Deaths from Fentanyl Abuse," *D Magazine*, December 6, 2018. https://healthcare.dmagazine.com/2018/12/05/ut-southwesterns-response-to-nurses-deaths-from-fentanyl-abuse/.

8. Christina Costantini and Darren Foster, "The Walter White of Wichita," *Fusion*, n.d. http://interactive.fusion.net/death-by-fentanyl/the-walter-white-of-wichita.html.

9. Mahony, "Stalking a 'Serial Killer' Narcotic."

10. "Understanding the Epidemic," Centers for Disease Control and Prevention, last reviewed March 19, 2020. https://www.cdc.gov/drugoverdose/epidemic/index.html.

11. *2018 National Drug Threat Assessment* (Washington, DC: Drug Enforcement Administration, 2018). https://www.dea.gov/sites/default/files/2018-11/DIR-032-18 2018 NDTA final low resolution.pdf.

12. Keegan Hamilton, "America's New Deadliest Drug Is Fentanyl," *Vice News*, August 30, 2016. https://www.vice.com/en_us/article/ev998e/americas-new-deadliest-drug-fentanyl.

13. *Fentanyl Remains the Most Significant Synthetic Opioid Threat and Poses the Greatest Threat to the Opioid User Market in the United States.* Report. (Washington, DC: Drug Enforcement Administration, 2018). https://ndews.umd.edu/sites/ndews.umd.edu/files/fentanyl-remains-most-significant-synthetic-opioid-threat-2018.pdf.

14. M. Jenkins, L. Diaz-Matos, M. Muchelli, and R. Rodriguez-Santana, "Fentanyl Testing and Reporting Project" (poster session presentation, Community Forum on Opioid Overdose Awareness and Prevention, Hartford, CT, May 30, 2018).

15. Office of the Chief Medical Examiner, "Connecticut Accidental Drug Intoxication Deaths" (data table). https://portal.ct.gov/-/media/OCME/Statistics/Calendar-Years-2012-to-2019-final.pdf?la=en.

16. Nicholas Rondinone, "One Dead after Three Suspected Overdoses in Hartford's North End, Fourth on Broad St.," *Hartford Courant*, December 06, 2018. https://www.courant.com/breaking-news/hc-hartford-overdoses-1102-20161101-story.html.

17. Martha Bebinger, "Fentanyl Adds a New Terror for People Abusing Opioids," NPR, April 6, 2017. https://www.npr.org/sections/health-shots/2017/04/06/521248448/fentanyl-adds-a-new-terror-for-people-abusing.

18. Glenn Burns, Rebecca T. DeRienz, Daniel D. Baker, Marcel Casavant, and Henry A. Spiller, "Could Chest Wall Rigidity Be a Factor in Rapid

Death from Illicit Fentanyl Abuse?," *Clinical Toxicology* 54, no. 5 (2016): 420–23. doi:10.3109/15563650.2016.1157722.

19. James B. Streisand, Peter L Bailey, Leon LeMaire, Michael A. Ashburn, Stephen D. Tarver, John Varvel, and Theodore H. Stanley, "Fentanyl-Induced Rigidity and Unconsciousness in Human Volunteers: Incidence, Duration, and Plasma Concentrations," *Anesthesiology* 78, no. 4 (1993): 629–34.

20. Mai-Lei Woo Kinshella, Tim Gauthier, and Mark Lysyshyn, "Rigidity, Dyskinesia and Other Atypical Overdose Presentations Observed at a Supervised Injection Site, Vancouver, Canada," *Harm Reduction Journal* 15, no. 1 (2018). doi:10.1186/s12954-018-0271-5.

21. Bryce Pardo, Jirka Taylor, Jonathan P. Caulkins, Beau Kilmer, Peter Reuter, and Bradley D. Stein, *The Future of Fentanyl and Other Synthetic Opioids* (Santa Monica, CA: RAND Corporation, 2019). https://www.rand.org/pubs/research_reports/RR3117.html.

22. "Ohio's Carfentanil Death Rate 21 Times Higher—yes, 2000%!— Than in Other States," Harm Reduction Ohio, August 6, 2018. https://www.harmreductionohio.org/deadly-mystery-ohio-carfentanil-death-rate-21-times-that-of-other-states/.

23. "Moscow Theater Hostage Crisis," Wikipedia, last edited February 26, 2020. https://en.wikipedia.org/wiki/Moscow_theater_hostage_crisis.

24. SarasotaSheriff, "Couple Discusses Heroin Overdoses and Potency Using Jail Phone," YouTube, February 27, 2017. https://www.youtube.com/watch?v=8ovFlbWrOyk.

25. "Nokomis Woman Charged in Overdose Death," 10 News, February 27, 2017. https://www.wtsp.com/article/news/local/nokomis-woman-charged-in-overdose-death/415504641.

26. "OxyContin Poster Children 15 Years Later," YouTube, September 09, 2012. https://www.youtube.com/watch?v=hwtSvHb_PRk; John Fauber and Ellen Gabler, "What Happened to the Poster Children of OxyContin?," *Milwaukee Journal Sentinel*, September 8, 2012. http://archive.jsonline.com/watchdog/watchdogreports/what-happened-to-the-poster-children-of-oxycontin-r65rolo-169056206.html.

Chapter 14. Responder Safety

1. "Fentanyl: A Real Threat to Law Enforcement," United States Department of Justice, October 5, 2016. https://www.justice.gov/opioid awareness/video/fentanyl-real-threat-law-enforcement.

2. *Fentanyl: A Briefing Guide for First Responders* (US Department of Justice, Drug Enforcement Administration, n.d.), 12. https://www.nvfc.org/wp-content/uploads/2018/03/Fentanyl-Briefing-Guide-for-First-Responders.pdf.

3. Peter Canning, "Fentanyl: A Briefing Guide for First Responders," *Medic Scribe*, January 19, 2019. http://www.medicscribe.com/2017/06/22 /fentanyl-a-briefing-guide-for-first-responders/.

4. Veronica Rocha, "1 Dead, 2 Others Hospitalized after Authorities Find White Powder in Santa Ana Apartment," *Los Angeles Times*, July 26, 2017. https://www.latimes.com/local/lanow/la-me-ln-drug-hazmat-santa -ana-20170726-story.html.

5. Zolan Kanno-Youngs and Corinne Ramey, "Fentanyl Isn't Just Deadly for Drug Users: Police Are Getting Sickened," *Wall Street Journal*, July 28, 2017. https://www.wsj.com/articles/an-american-scourge-fentanyl -is-now-stinging-law-enforcement-1501234203.

6. Jeremy Samuel Faust, "The Viral Story about the Cop Who Over-dosed by Touching Fentanyl Is Nonsense," *Slate*, June 28, 2017. https://amp .slate.com/articles/health_and_science/medical_examiner/2017/06 /toxicologists_explain_the_medical_impossibility_of_overdosing_by _touching.html.

7. David Anderson, "Md. Officer Recounts Exposure to Heroin, Fentanyl on Overdose Call," *EMS World*, May 28, 2017. https://www.emsworld.com /news/12338852/md-officer-recounts-exposure-to-heroin-fentanyl-on -overdose-call.

8. Jill Harmacinski McClatchy, "Mass. Fire Chief Seeks Improved Protocols for Opioid Overdoses," *EMS World*, July 31, 2017. https://www .emsworld.com/news/218325/mass-fire-chief-seeks-improved-protocols -opioid-overdoses.

9. *ACMT and AACT Position Statement: Preventing Occupational Fentanyl and Fentanyl Analog Exposure to Emergency Responders*, American College of Medical Toxicology, n.d. https://www.acmt.net/_Library/Positions /Fentanyl_PPE_Emergency_Responders_.pdf.

10. Nicholas Rondinone, "Acting Head of DEA Rosenberg Spends Last Day at Yale," *Hartford Courant*, December 12, 2018. https://www.courant .com/health/hc-news-dea-rosenberg-yale-keynote-20170928-story.html.

11. Jon B. Cole and Lewis S. Nelson, "Controversies and Carfentanil: We Have Much to Learn about the Present State of Opioid Poisoning," *American Journal of Emergency Medicine* 35, no. 11 (2017): 1743–45.

12. Steve Birr, "Officers Hospitalized after Becoming Dizzy and Feeling 'a Tingling Sensation' at Scene of Fatal Fentanyl Overdose," *Daily Caller*, September 2, 2018. https://dailycaller.com/2018/09/02/police-fentanyl -exposure-massachusetts/.

13. Aaron Moody, "Cops Left Dizzy and Numb after Exposure to Mysterious Substance during NC Drug Search," *Raleigh News and Observer*, August 7, 2018. https://www.newsobserver.com/news/state/north-carolina /article216255660.html.

14. "Advisory: Fentanyl Safety Recommendations for First Respond-ers," Office of National Drug Control Policy, White House, n.d. https://www.whitehouse.gov/ondcp/key-issues/fentanyl/.

15. US Customs and Border Protection, *Fentanyl: The Real Deal*, YouTube, August 30, 2018. https://www.youtube.com/watch?v=6Yc9lSaSKls&feature=youtu.be.

Chapter 16. Partners

1. Emilie Munson, "In Purdue Pharma Opioid Fight, CT Turns Atten-tion to Doctors," *Connecticut Post*, April 24, 2019. https://www.ctpost.com/politics/article/In-Purdue-Pharma-opioid-fight-CT-turns-attention-13789962.php.

2. A complaint was filed on June 13, 2018, in Suffolk Superior Court in the lawsuit *Massachusetts v. Purdue Pharma*: https://www.mass.gov/files/documents/2018/06/12/Purdue%20Complaint%20FILED.pdf.

Chapter 17.   Mental Health

1. *Number of Opioid-Related Overdose Deaths, All Intents by City/Town, MA Residents, January 2012–December 2016* (Massachusetts Department of Public Health, May 2017). https://www.mass.gov/files/documents/2017/08/31/town-by-town-listings-may-2017.pdf.

2. Martha Bebinger, "How Many Opioid Overdoses Are Suicides?," NPR, March 15, 2018. https://www.npr.org/sections/health-shots/2018/03/15/591577807/how-many-opioid-overdoses-are-suicides.

3. Bebinger, "How Many Opioid Overdoses Are Suicides?"

4. Alix Spiegel, "What Vietnam Taught Us about Breaking Bad Habits," NPR, January 2, 2012. https://www.npr.org/sections/health-shots/2012/01/02/144431794/what-vietnam-taught-us-about-breaking-bad-habits.

5. Bruce K. Alexander, "Rat Park. Addiction: The View from Rat Park," personal website, 2010. http://brucekalexander.com/articles-speeches/rat-park/148-addiction-the-view-from-rat-park.

6. Adi Jaffe, "Addiction, Connection and the Rat Park Study," *Psychol-ogy Today*, August 14, 2015. https://www.psychologytoday.com/us/blog/all-about-addiction/201508/addiction-connection-and-the-rat-park-study.

7. Raychelle Cassad Lohmann, "Childhood Sexual Trauma and Addiction," *Psychology Today*, January 26, 2018. https://www.psychologytoday.com/us/blog/teen-angst/201801/childhood-sexual-trauma-and-addiction.

Chapter 18. Age

1. Peter Canning, Charles McKay, Suzanne Doyon, Elizabeth Laska, Katherine Hart, and Richard Kamin, "Coordinated Surveillance of Opioid

Overdoses in Hartford, Connecticut: A Pilot Project," *Connecticut Medicine* 83, no. 6 (2019): 293–99.

Chapter 19. The War on Drugs

1. "A Brief History of the Drug War," Drug Policy Alliance, n.d. http://www.drugpolicy.org/issues/brief-history-drug-war.

2. "2018: Crime in the United States," Federal Bureau of Investigation: Uniform Crime Reporting, n.d. https://ucr.fbi.gov/crime-in-the-u.s/2018 /crime-in-the-u.s.-2018/topic-pages/persons-arrested.

3. Nick Wing, "Drug Dealer Sentenced to 20 Years for Murder after Customer's Fatal Overdose," *HuffPost*, April 13, 2017. https://www.huffpost .com/entry/fentanyl-dealer-murder-conviction_n_58efafdee4b0b9e98 48a33fa.

4. John Temple, "DEA Secretly OKs Killer Quantities of Oxy and Morphine," *Daily Beast*, October 21, 2015. https://www.thedailybeast.com /dea-secretly-oks-killer-quantities-of-oxy-and-morphine.

5. Nicholas Rondinone, "After Two Deaths, Feds Charge Alleged Hartford Heroin Dealers," *Hartford Courant*, April 25, 2016. https://www .courant.com/health/hc-hartford-kd-arrest-follow-0426-20160425-story .html.

6. Nicholas Rondinone, "Hartford Man Gets 6 Years after Pleading Guilty to Selling Heroin Linked to Two Deadly Overdoses," *Hartford Courant*, April 25, 2017. https://www.courant.com/breaking-news/hc-hartford-heroin -dealer-sentenced-20170425-story.html.

7. Bureau of Justice Statistics, *Drug Use and Dependence, State and Federal Prisoners, 2004*, revised January 19, 2007. http://www.bjs.gov /content/pub/pdf/dudsfp04.pdf.

8. Meghan Peterson, Josiah Rich, Alexandria Macmadu, Ashley Q. Truong, Traci C. Green, Leo Beletsky, Kimberly Pognon, and Lauren Brinkley-Rubinstein, "'One Guy Goes to Jail, Two People Are Ready to Take His Spot': Perspectives on Drug-Induced Homicide Laws among Incarcerated Individuals," *International Journal of Drug Policy* 70 (2019): 47–53.

9. Ingrid A. Binswanger, Marc F. Stern, Richard A. Deyo, Patrick J. Heagerty, Allen Cheadle, Joann G. Elmore, and Thomas D. Koepsell, "Release from Prison—a High Risk of Death for Former Inmates," *New England Journal of Medicine* 356, no. 2 (2007): 157–65.

10. Traci C. Green, Jennifer Clarke, Lauren Brinkley-Rubinstein, Brandon D. L. Marshall, Nicole Alexander-Scott, Rebecca Boss, and Josiah D. Rich, "Postincarceration Fatal Overdoses after Implementing Medications for Addiction Treatment in a Statewide Correctional System," *JAMA Psychiatry* 75, no. 4 (2018): 405–7.

11. Timothy Williams, "Opioid Users Are Filling Jails. Why Don't Jails Treat Them?," *New York Times*, August 4, 2017. https://www.nytimes.com/2017/08/04/us/heroin-addiction-jails-methadone-suboxone-treatment.html.

12. Matt Ormseth, "After Battling Addiction, Sarah Howroyd Started HOPE," *Hartford Courant*, June 29, 2017. https://www.courant.com/news/connecticut/hc-hometown-hero-sarah-howroyd-20170629-story.html.

13. "For Addicts and Their Friends, Families, and Caregivers," Gloucester Police Department, accessed August 18, 2019. https://gloucesterpd.com/addicts/.

Chapter 21. Children

1. "Advertising and Promotion of Alcohol and Tobacco Products to Youth," American Public Health Association. https://www.apha.org/policies-and-advocacy/public-health-policy-statements/policy-database/2014/07/29/10/58/advertising-and-promotion-of-alcohol-and-tobacco-products-to-youth; Paul M. Fischer, Meyer P. Schwartz, John W. Richards, Adam O. Goldstein, and Tina H. Rojas, "Brand Logo Recognition by Children Aged 3 to 6 Years: Mickey Mouse and Old Joe the Camel," *JAMA* 266, no. 22 (1991): 3145-48.

2. Jean H. Lee, "R. J. Reynolds Agrees to Pay $10 Million in Joe Camel Lawsuit," AP News, September 9, 1997. https://www.apnews.com/ce9e3e9c7595bae5034193112a75bb7e.

Chapter 22. Community Naloxone

1. Northbay MDS, "Harm Reduction: Dealing with the Prevalence of Opiates and Other 'Hard' Drugs," December 1, 2014. https://northbaymds.blogspot.com/2014/12/harm-reduction-dealing-with-prevalence.html.

2. Heather Mack, "Cartooning on Clarion Alley to Prevent Overdoses," *Mission Local*, September 23, 2013. https://missionlocal.org/2013/09/cartooning-on-clarion-alley-to-prevent-overdoses/.

3. Jennifer Doleac and Anita Mukherjee, "The Moral Hazard of Lifesaving Innovations: Naloxone Access, Opioid Abuse, and Crime." Archived at SSRN: http://dx.doi.org/10.2139/ssrn.3135264.

4. Jermaine D. Jones, Aimee Campbell, Verena E. Metz, and Sandra D. Comer, "No Evidence of Compensatory Drug Use Risk Behavior among Heroin Users after Receiving Take-Home Naloxone," *Addictive Behaviors* 71 (2017): 104-6.

5. Rebecca McDonald and John Strang, "Are Take-Home Naloxone Programmes Effective? Systematic Review Utilizing Application of the Bradford Hill Criteria," *Addiction* 111, no. 7 (2016): 1177-87.

Chapter 23. Safe-Injection Site

1. Connecticut Department of Public Heath, Office of Emergency Medical Services, unpublished data furnished to the author, covering 2015–2016.

2. Peter Canning, Charles McKay, Suzanne Doyon, Elizabeth Laska, Katherine Hart, and Richard Kamin, "Coordinated Surveillance of Opioid Overdoses in Hartford, Connecticut: A Pilot Project," *Connecticut Medicine* 83, no. 6 (June/July 2019): 293–99.

3. "Insite—Supervised Consumption Site," Vancouver Coastal Health. http://www.vch.ca/Locations-Services/result?res_id=964.

4. "Insite User Statistics," Vancouver Coastal Health. http://www.vch .ca/public-health/harm-reduction/supervised-consumption-sites/insite -user-statistics.

5. "Onsite—Detox Facility," Vancouver Coastal Health. http://www.vch .ca/Locations-Services/result?res_id=1397.

6. Brandon D. L. Marshall, Michael Jay Milloy, Evan Wood, Julio S. G. Montaner, and Thomas Kerr, "Reduction in Overdose Mortality after the Opening of North America's First Medically Supervised Safer Injecting Facility: A Retrospective Population-Based Study," *The Lancet* 377, no. 9775 (2011): 1429–37.

7. Kora DeBeck, Thomas Kerr, Lorna Bird, Ruth Zhang, David Marsh, Mark Tyndall, Julio Montaner, and Evan Wood, "Injection Drug Use Cessation and Use of North America's First Medically Supervised Safer Injecting Facility," *Drug and Alcohol Dependence* 113, nos. 2–3 (2011): 172–76.

8. Evan Wood, Mark W. Tyndall, Ruth Zhang, Julio S. G. Montaner, and Thomas Kerr, "Rate of Detoxification Service Use and Its Impact among a Cohort of Supervised Injecting Facility Users," *Addiction* 102, no. 6 (2007): 916–19.

9. Amos Irwin, Ehsan Jozaghi, Brian W. Weir, Sean T. Allen, Andrew Lindsay, and Susan G. Sherman, "Mitigating the Heroin Crisis in Baltimore, MD, USA: A Cost-Benefit Analysis of a Hypothetical Supervised Injection Facility," *Harm Reduction Journal* 14, no. 1 (2017): article no. 29. doi:10.1186/s12954-017-0153-2.

10. Elana Gordon, "What's the Evidence That Supervised Drug Injection Sites Save Lives?," NPR, September 7, 2018. https://www.npr.org /sections/health-shots/2018/09/07/645609248/whats-the-evidence-that -supervised-drug-injection-sites-save-lives.

11. Leo Beletsky, Corey S. Davis, Evan Anderson, and Scott Burris, "The Law (and Politics) of Safe Injection Facilities in the United States," *American Journal of Public Health* 98, no. 2 (2008): 231–37.

12. Bobby Allyn, "Justice Department Promises Crackdown on Supervised Injection Facilities," NPR, August 30, 2018. https://www.npr.org

/sections/health-shots/2018/08/30/642735759/justice-department
-promises-crackdown-on-supervised-injection-sites.

13. Erin Schumaker, "Former Philadelphia Mayor Calls Approval of
Safe-Injection Site 'Hugely Important.'" ABC News, October 3, 2019.
https://abcnews.go.com/US/philadelphia-mayor-calls-approval-safe
-injection-site-hugely/story?id=66034723.

14. Johns Hopkins University Bloomberg School of Public Health,
"Support Increases When Opioid 'Safe Consumption Sites' Called 'Overdose Prevention Sites,'" *Medical Xpress*, August 8, 2018. https://www.jhsph
.edu/news/news-releases/2018/support-increases-when-opioid-safe
-consumption-sites-called-overdose-prevention-sites.html.

15. Mary Clare Kennedy and Thomas Kerr, "Overdose Prevention in the
United States: A Call for Supervised Injection Sites," *American Journal of
Public Health* 107, no. 1 (January 1, 2017): 42–43.

16. Anna Gorman, "Needle Exchanges Can Now Get Federal Funding,"
Kaiser Health News, February 17, 2016. https://khn.org/news/needle
-exchanges-can-now-get-federal-funding/.

17. North American Syringe Exchange Network. https://www.nasen
.org/map/.

18. Richard L. Vogt, Mark C. Breda, Don C. Des Jarlais, Sena Gates, and
Peter Whiticar, "Hawaii's Statewide Syringe Exchange Program," *American Journal of Public Health* 88, no. 9 (1998): 1403–4.

19. Holly Hagan, James P. McGough, Hanne Thiede, Sharon Hopkins,
Jeffrey Duchin, and E. Russell Alexander, "Reduced Injection Frequency
and Increased Entry and Retention in Drug Treatment Associated with
Needle-Exchange Participation in Seattle Drug Injectors," *Journal of
Substance Abuse Treatment* 19, no. 3 (2000): 247–52.

20. Peter Canning, "Insight: I See What Heroin Does. Let People Shoot
Up Safely," *Hartford Courant*, December 6, 2018. https://www.courant
.com/opinion/op-ed/hc-insight-let-heroin-users-shoot-up-safely-20180730
-story.html.

21. "Insight: 5 Things to Know about Opioid Addiction," *Hartford
Courant*, December 6, 2018. https://www.courant.com/opinion/op-ed/hc
-insight-5-things-about-heroin-20180801-story.html.

Chapter 24. Cut

1. "Carfentanil Unexpectedly Returns to Ohio Drug Supply; Overdose
Deaths Surge," Harm Reduction Ohio, May 24, 2019. https://www.harmr
eductionohio.org/carfentanil-unexpectedly-returns-to-ohios-drug
-supply/.

Chapter 25. Danger Ahead

1. *Counterfeit Prescription Pills Containing Fentanyls: A Global Threat.* Report, Drug Enforcement Administration, July 2016. https://www.dea.gov/sites/default/files/docs/Counterfeit%2520Prescription%2520Pills.pdf.

2. *2018 National Drug Assessment.* Report, US Department of Justice, Drug Enforcement Administration, 2018. https://www.dea.gov/documents/2018/10/02/2018-national-drug-threat-assessment-ndta.

3. Nicholas Rondinone, "Deadly Fentanyl Disguised as Prescription Pills," *Hartford Courant,* July 3, 2017. https://www.courant.com/news/connecticut/hc-fentanyl-as-pills-20170703-story.html.

4. Daniella Silva, "Prince Died after Taking Fake Vicodin Laced with Fentanyl, Prosecutor Says," NBCNews.com, April 19, 2018. https://www.nbcnews.com/news/us-news/no-criminal-charges-prince-s-overdose-death-prosecutor-announces-n867491.

Chapter 26. The Bakery

1. "Heroin Island, NYC," *Drugs, Inc.,* season 7, episode 10, aired November 18, 2015, on National Geographic Channel.

Chapter 27. Call of Duty

1. "Poster Project," Today I Matter, n.d. https://www.todayimatter.org/poster-project.html.

2. "Hippocratic Oath," *Wikipedia,* last edited March 27, 2020. https://en.wikipedia.org/wiki/Hippocratic_Oath.

3. "Daphne Willis—Somebody's Someone," YouTube, February 17, 2017. https://youtu.be/uGgN9vMPUn8.

Chapter 28. Plateau

1. *Merriam-Webster,* s.v. "plateau (*n.*)," "plateau (*v.*)," accessed April 10, 2020. https://www.merriam-webster.com/dictionary/plateau.

2. Emily Sullivan, "Opioid Deaths May Be Starting to Plateau, HHS Chief Says," NPR, October 24, 2018. https://www.npr.org/2018/10/24/660089369/opioid-deaths-are-starting-to-plateau-u-s-health-chief-says.

3. "US Drug Overdose Death Rates and Totals over Time," Wikipedia, last edited on February 14, 2020. https://en.wikipedia.org/wiki/US_drug_overdose_death_rates_and_totals_over_time.

4. "Accidental Drug Related Deaths, 2012–2019," CT.gov. https://data.ct.gov/Health-and-Human-Services/Accidental-Drug-Related-Deaths-2012-2019/rybz-nyjw.

5. *Merriam-Webster,* s.v. "ensnare (*v.*)," accessed April 10, 2020. https://www.merriam-webster.com/dictionary/ensnare.

6. *CT Bar Association and CT Bar Foundation Opioid Conference at Quinnipiac University School of Law* (video), Connecticut Network, November 9, 2018. http://ct-n.com/ctnplayer.asp?odID=15751.

7. "Accidental Drug Related Deaths, 2012–2019," CT.gov. https://data .ct.gov/Health-and-Human-Services/Accidental-Drug-Related-Deaths -2012-2019/rybz-nyjw.

Chapter 29. State Capitol

1. Lydia Gerike, "Three More Overdose Deaths in Hartford Bring Week's Total to 10 as Count Runs Far Ahead of Last Year's," *Hartford Courant*, June 10, 2019. https://www.courant.com/community/hartford /hc-news-opioid-overdose-death-roundtable-20190610-fvqz5kqru5gwze fitqmepn5hcm-story.html.

2. Erin E. Krebs, Amy Gravely, Sean Nugent, Agnes C. Jensen, Beth DeRonne, Elizabeth S. Goldsmith, Kurt Kroenke, Matthew J. Bair, and Siamak Noorbaloochi, "Effect of Opioid vs Nonopioid Medications on Pain-Related Function in Patients with Chronic Back Pain or Hip or Knee Osteoarthritis Pain: The SPACE Randomized Clinical Trial," *JAMA* 319, no. 9 (2018): 872–82; Kai S. Tsang, Jon Page, and Paul Mackenney, "Can Intravenous Paracetamol Reduce Opioid Use in Preoperative Hip Fracture Patients?," *Orthopedics* 36, no. 2 (2013): 20–24.

3. Gaëlle Faure, "Why Doctors Are Giving Heroin to Heroin Addicts," *Time*, September 28, 2009. http://content.time.com/time/health/article /0,8599,1926160,00.html.

INDEX

personal protective equipment (PPE), 146, 147, 148, 150
peyote, 195
pharmaceutical companies: lobbying activities, 86; marketing practices, 141–42; responsibility for opioid crisis, 2, 78–80, 86, 91–92, 127–28, 141–42, 189
Picard, Dan, 27
Pino, Raul, 260
pleasure, 42–43, 43–44
Pope Francis, 99–100
Porter, Jane, 85
Prince (rock singer), 240
prisons. *See* jails and prisons
Proxmire, William, 259
Purdue Pharma, 78–79, 85, 88, 92, 127–28, 141, 166–67

Quaaludes, 91

racial discrimination, 253–54
RAND Corporation, 139
recovery: harm reduction and, 111–12; readiness for, 59–60; social support for, 173
recovery coaches, 116–17, 192
rehabilitation, relapse after, 114–16, 121, 155; after incarceration, 63; tolerance and, 31–32, 188–89, 250–51
reward center, of brain, 6, 41, 42–43, 46, 62, 66
"Rhetoric of Recovery Advocacy: An Essay on the Power of Language, The" (White), 49–50
Rick, Herschel, 85
Rigby, Robert, 140
Riley, Jack, 143–44
R. J. Reynolds, 199
Rosen, Jeffrey, 223
Rosenberg, Chuck, 144, 149
Rosenstein, Rod, 223
Russia, 148

Sabin, Bryan, 45, 99, 169, 191, 229
Safehouse, 223
safe-injection sites, 112, 138–39, 212–27, 265; cost-benefit analysis, 220–21; heroin houses, 214–16, 217;

opposition to, 222–24, 225; overdose rates and, 220–21
safe-injection techniques, 201
St. Francis Hospital and Medical Center, 34, 39, 63–64, 117, 125, 193, 194, 262; Suboxone program, 59–60, 271
saline bullets, 118
scene safety, 143–50
Schweitzer, Albert, 82–83
sex workers, 230–32, 266
shame: as barrier to recovery, 48–49, 57; opioids as escape from, 74, 172–73; stigmatization-related, 41, 47, 48 10, 50, 257
Smith, Cassandra, 263
Sneed, Jerry, 17, 19–22, 34, 37, 63, 101, 102, 151
social isolation, 173
Society of Addiction Medicine, 41
Spanos, Alan, 78
speedballs, 137–38
stereotypes of drug users, 179
sternal rub, 66, 158, 237
stigma, of drug user, 1–2, 10, 23, 47–54, 253, 265; effect on addiction treatment, 77; effect on families, 41, 77; effect on recovery, 50–51; by first responders, 25–29; language of, 49–51; three Ds of, 48
Suboxone, 28, 59–60, 61–62, 64, 153, 154, 170–71, 190; availability, 117, 264–65; naloxone content, 170
suicide, 36, 167, 172–78

temptation to use opioids, 194–98
THC, 230
Today I Matter project, 252–53
tolerance, 43, 87–88, 116, 127; after abstinence, 209; after incarceration, 190–91; after rehabilitation, 31–32, 188–89, 250–51; drug dealers' monitoring of, 202
Toradol, 88–89, 264
Tylenol, 261
Tyson, LaToya, 225–26

University of Connecticut John Dempsey Hospital, 107